Assisted Reproduction

Progress in Research and Practice

Advances
in Reproductive
Endocrinology

VOLUME 7

Assisted Reproduction

Progress in Research and Practice

Edited by RW Shaw

The Parthenon Publishing Group

International Publishers in Medicine, Science & Technology

Casterton Hall, Carnforth,
Lancs, LA6 2LA, UK

One Blue Hill Plaza, Pearl River,
New York 10965, USA

Published in the UK by
The Parthenon Publishing Group Limited
Casterton Hall, Carnforth,
Lancs, LA6 2LA, England

Published in the USA by
The Parthenon Publishing Group Inc.
One Blue Hill Plaza
PO Box 1564, Pearl River,
New York 10965, USA

British Library Cataloguing in Publication Data

Assisted Reproduction: Progress in
Research and Practice. – (Advances in
Reproductive Endocrinology; Vol.7)
 I. Shaw, Robert W.   II. Series
 618.178059

 ISBN 1-85070-679-4

Library of Congress Cataloging-in-Publication Data

Assisted reproduction: progress in research and practice / edited by R.W. Shaw.
   p.   cm. — (Advances in reproductive endocrinology: v. 7)
 Proceeding of a workshop held in St. John's College, Cambridge, UK in July 1994.
 Includes bibiographical references and index.
 ISBN   1-85070-679-4
   1. Fertilization in vitro, Human — congresses.   2. Human reproductive
technology — Congresses.   I. Shaw, Robert W. (Robert Wayne)   II. Series.
   [DNLM: 1. Fertilization in vitro — congresses.   2. Reproduction Techniques —
congresses.   W1 AD83S v.7 1995 / WQ 205 A8402 1995]
RG135.A86   1995
618.1'78—dc20
DNLM/DLC   95-15486
for Library of Congress   CIP

Composition by Keele University Press, England
Printed and Bound in Great Britain by
Butler and Tanner Ltd, Frome and London

Contents

List of principal contributors

N. Amso
Department of Obstetrics and
   Gynaecology
Queen Elizabeth Hospital
Sheriff Hill
Gateshead
Tyne & Wear NE9 6SX
UK

R.G. Forman
UMDS
Guy's and St Thomas's Medical
   and Dental School
Division of Obstetrics and
   Gynaecology
St Thomas's Hospital
Lambeth Palace Road
London SE1 7EH
UK

R.K. Goswamy
The Churchill Clinic and IVF
   Centre
80 Lambeth Road
London SE1 7PW
UK

S. Green
NURTURE
Department of Obstetrics and
   Gynaecology
Floor B East Block
University Hospital
Queen's Medical Centre
Nottingham NG7 2UH
UK

L. Gregory
Unit for Assisted Reproduction
University Hospital of Wales
Heath Park
Cardiff CF4 4XW
UK

A.H. Handyside
Institute of Obstetrics and
   Gynaecology
Royal Postgraduate Medical
   School
Hammersmith Hospital
Du Cane Road
London W12 0NN
UK

H.J. Leese
The Department of Biology
University of York
Heslington
York YO1 5DD
UK

E.A. Lenton
University of Sheffield
Department of Obstetrics and
  Gynaecology
Jessops Hospital for Women
Sheffield S1 7RE
UK

B.A. Lieberman
Manchester Fertility Services Ltd
Manchester BUPA Hospital
Russell House
Russell Road
Whalley Range
Manchester M16 8AJ
UK

P.L. Matson
Department of Reproductive
  Medicine
St Mary's Hospital
Whitworth Park
Manchester M13 0JH
UK

R.W. Shaw
Department of Obstetrics and
  Gynaecology
University of Wales College of
  Medicine
Heath Park
Cardiff CF4 4XN
UK

Foreword

The techniques of *in vitro* fertilization (IVF) have been in practice in the United Kingdom on a wide basis for the last decade. The techniques employed today are very different to those first pioneered by Edwards and Steptoe in the late 1970s, but still embrace underlying basic principles.

Success rates, in terms of ongoing pregnancy rates per embryo transfer, have improved from 5% to around 20% (currently) for most centres despite, in many instances, a reduction in the number of embryos transferred – currently limited to three, under the Human Fertilisation and Embryology Authority's regulation.

Many new techniques have been developed to widen the application of assisted conception methods to a much broader group of infertile couples. Perhaps one of the most significant developments has been that of intracytoplasmic sperm injection (ICSI).

Clearly there is still room for improvement in identifying appropriate methods of ovarian stimulation: embryo assessment; increased implantation rates; appropriate methods of cryopreserving gametes and embryos; and refinement in the selection of couples for more complex variations of IVF treatment.

The chapters in this seventh volume of Advances in Reproductive Endocrinology are the results of a workshop on Assisted Reproduction held in St John's College, Cambridge in July, 1994. At this workshop, a number of areas within this field of research were reviewed by recognized national and international experts. The meeting was sponsored by an Education Department grant from Zeneca Pharma (UK) to whom we are most grateful.

It is hoped that the contents will add some insight for clinicians, embryologists and biologists into current research and progress in this continually expanding field of assisted conception.

Professor Robert W. Shaw
Department of Obstetrics and Gynaecology
University of Wales College of Medicine
Cardiff
February, 1995

1

Anomalies of human pre-implantation development *in vitro*

A. H. Handyside and K. Hardy

INTRODUCTION

Pregnancy rates after *in vitro* fertilization (IVF) remain low. In the UK, average pregnancy rates per treatment cycle had been increasing (from 11 to 17% between 1985 and 1990) but now appear to have reached a plateau (19% in 1992)[1]. Nevertheless, in centres that have had more experience, excluding male infertility and women over 40 years of age, pregnancy and live birth rates of at least 25 and 20%, respectively, are consistently achieved and cumulative rates are close to those resulting from normal conception in fertile couples. This suggests that the limiting factor may now be embryo quality, a view supported by the poor development of human embryos to the advanced pre-implantation stages *in vitro*. Careful examination of surplus, normally fertilized embryos has revealed a high incidence of a variety of cytoplasmic, nuclear and chromosomal abnormalities even at early cleavage stages; only about half reach the blastocyst stage and a proportion of blastocysts also appear to be abnormal.

WHOLE EMBRYO ARREST

Almost half of embryos classified as normally fertilized (based on the identification of two pronuclei 16–18 h after insemination) arrest and fail to develop to the blastocyst stage *in vitro*[2]. Combining the results from a number of studies, analysis of the stage of developmental arrest indicates that human embryos arrest at all stages from the 1-cell to morula stages (Figure 1). One possible cause of the poor development *in vitro* is suboptimal culture conditions. The simple culture media used routinely for IVF are based on those that have been used successfully in other species, particularly mice, and they may not be optimal or sufficient for development beyond the early stages *in vitro*. There is increasing evidence, in both the human and other animal species, that subtle alterations in the composition of the culture medium can produce significant improvements in embryo development.

Cleavage stage block

Embryos from a variety of mammalian species block at specific cleavage stages during *in vitro* culture. Mouse zygotes from outbred and many inbred strains arrest at the 2-cell stage ('2-cell block'); the hamster at the 2-cell stage; the cow and sheep at the 8- to 16-cell stage; and the pig at the 4- to 8-cell stage[3]. Bolton and colleagues[4] found that the majority of surplus human embryos which arrest do so between the 4- and 8-cell stages. In all the aforementioned species, this block coincides with the stage at which the embryo is undergoing the transition from control by maternal RNA laid down during oogenesis to embryonic control, when transcriptional activation of the embryonic genome is switched on[5–8]. The failure of embryos to develop beyond the block is thought to be a consequence of their being particularly sensitive to sub-optimal culture conditions during this period. Evidence for this has been provided by experiments in which altering the composition of the culture medium has overcome the developmental block. In several species, including mouse[9,10], hamster[11], rat[12] and sheep[13], glucose has been demonstrated to be inhibitory during early cleavage, for reasons which are not fully understood. In the mouse, the combination of omitting glucose, increasing the lactate:pyruvate ratio and supplementing the medium with glutamine overcomes the 2-cell block[9]. In the hamster, the beneficial effects of removing glucose are potentiated by omitting phosphate[14,15]. We have also recently demonstrated that glucose may be inhibitory in the human. Removal of glucose from day 2 onwards, although not increasing the proportion of embryos developing to the blastocyst stage, significantly increases the numbers of trophectoderm cells at this stage[16].

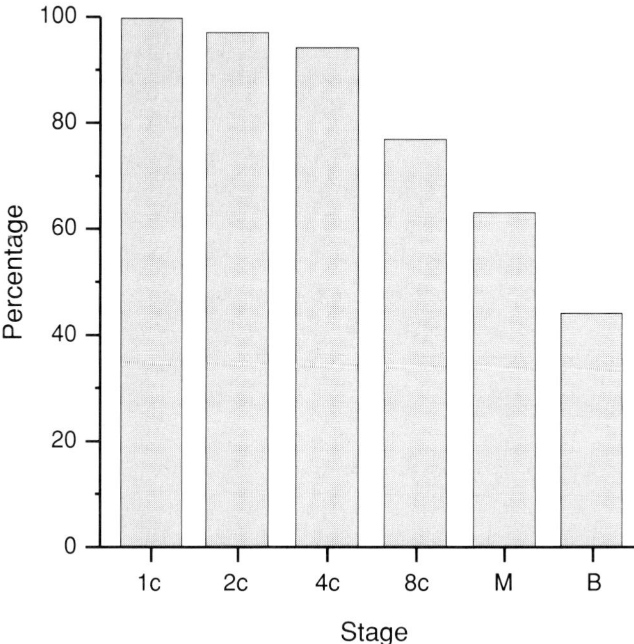

Figure 1 Development of 609 surplus human embryos *in vitro* between days 1 and 6 following oocyte retrieval and insemination; M, morula; B, blastocyst

In addition to glutamine, other amino acids (particularly glycine and taurine) are also critical for overcoming cleavage stage arrest in other species, including the hamster, allowing a large proportion of embryos to develop to the blastocyst stage (reviewed by Bavister and McKiernan[17]). Interestingly, these amino acids are found in high concentrations in the reproductive tract of various species, and also in the amino acid pools of pre-implantation mouse embryos themselves[18]. Furthermore, the development of blocking and non-blocking strains of mouse embryos to the blastocyst stage and cell numbers are significantly improved by the addition of ion chelators[19–22] or non-essential amino acids[23]. As yet, the physiological roles of high levels of these amino acids in reproductive tract fluid and the embryo are unknown, although several have been proposed, including:

(1) Metabolic substrates for energy production (several amino acids can indirectly enter the tricarboxylic acid cycle and glutamine is known to be used as a substrate).

(2) Anabolic substrates for protein synthesis.

(3) Organic osmoregulators.

(4) Chelators of heavy metal ions which would otherwise be detrimental.

(5) Regulators of intracellular pH (for example, mouse embryos lack the Na^+/H^+ antiporter which is important in reducing intracellular acid load; glycine and taurine could export excess intracellular protons).

PARTIAL EMBRYO ARREST

A feature of human pre-implantation development *in vitro* is the prevalence of morphological abnormalities, including uneven cleavage, cytoplasmic fragmentation and degenerate cells (Figure 2). Even at late pre-implantation stages various gross abnormalities can be seen, including morulae and blastocysts with excluded blastomeres, large cells in the blastocoele cavity and multiple cavities. The presence of excluded cells and large cells in the blastocoele cavity suggests that, during cleavage, one or more cells cease division and persist as cells which are unincorporated in the developing embryo.

Cytoplasmic, nuclear and chromosomal abnormalities at cleavage stages

Labelling of embryos with polynucleotide-specific fluorochromes, such as Hoechst 33342, reveals a high prevalence of nuclear abnormalities which are not commonly seen in embryos of other species such as the mouse (Figure 3). These abnormalities include binucleate and anucleate cells, and cells with multiple or fragmenting nuclei[24, 25]. Binucleate cells are common; at early cleavage stages, 17% of embryos have at least one binucleate blastomere, and by the 8- to 16-cell stage, 65% of embryos have between one and six binucleate blastomeres. The incidence of anucleate blastomeres is also high, particularly in embryos of poor morphology.

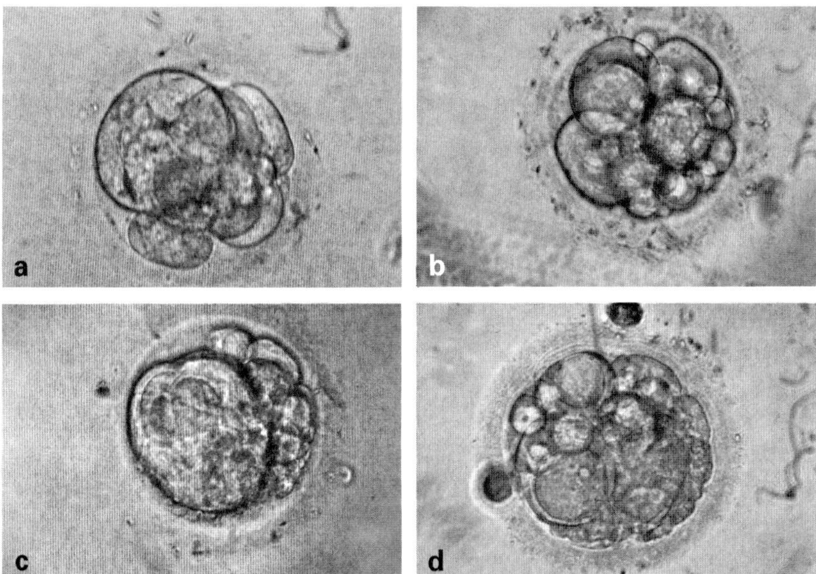

Figure 2 Morphological abnormalities of human embryos developing *in vitro*: (a) uneven cleavage, (b) cytoplasmic fragmentation, (c) a morula with excluded cells and (d) intracellular vacuolation

Blastomeres with fragmenting or multiple nuclei are relatively uncommon. Binucleate cells are frequently larger than the other, mononucleate cells within the embryo. Measuring these cells, and assigning them to cleavage stages, indicates that binucleate cells have arrested at earlier cleavage divisions, while the mononucleate cells have progressed through cleavage.

Chromosomal mosaicism

Multicolour fluorescent *in situ* hybridization (FISH) with different chromosome-specific probes now allows the analysis of the majority of interphase nuclei from individual embryos. These studies have demonstrated that human embryos *in vitro* are often mosaic for cells with aneuploidies involving several chromosomes[26, 27]. Clearly, these chromosomal abnormalities must arise during early cleavage and their chaotic nature is reminiscent of transformed cells in culture. Cell cycle checkpoints,

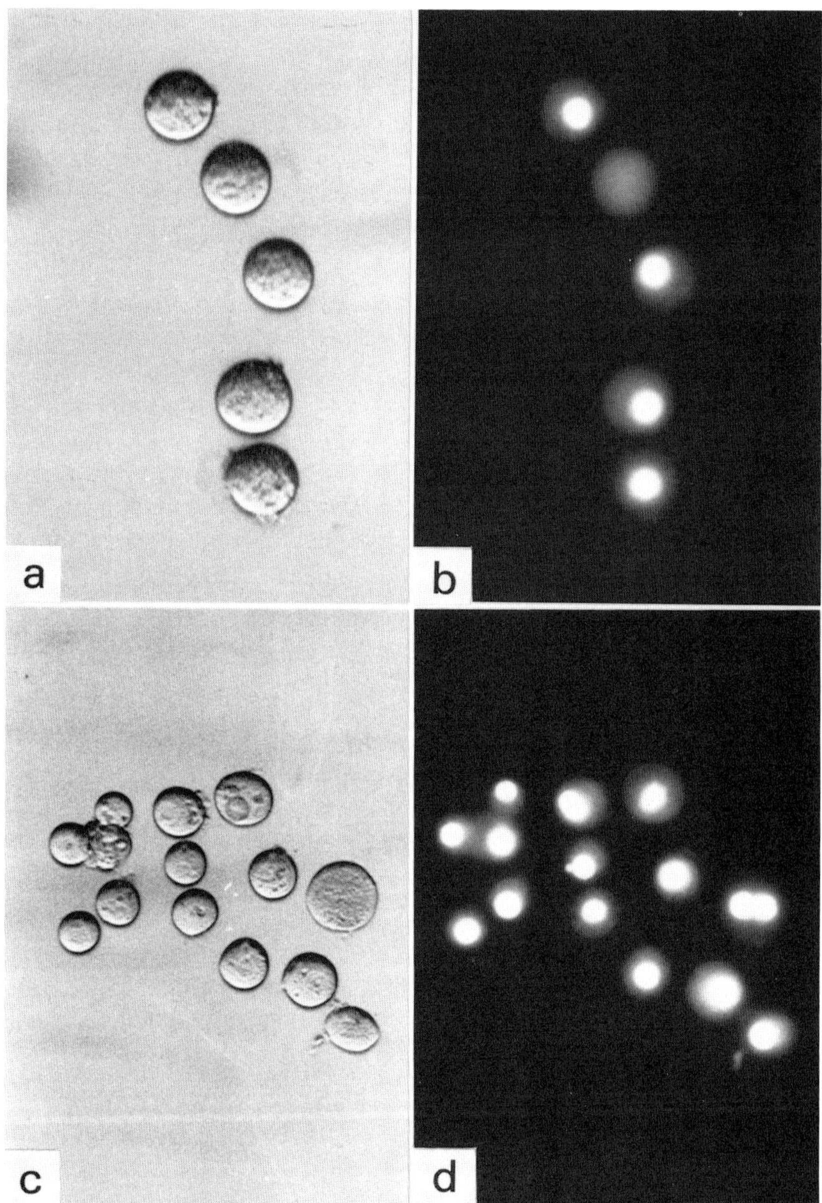

Figure 3 Common nuclear abnormalities in disaggregated blastomeres from cleavage stage human embryos developing *in vitro* stained with the DNA fluorochrome Hoechst 33342: (a,b) anucleate blastomere, and (c,d) binucleate blastomere

first identified in yeast, would normally protect cells from genetic damage by ensuring that successive phases of the cell cycle are completed before the next is initiated[28, 29]. For example, there is a checkpoint that prevents mitosis proceeding before completion of chromosomal segregation. In transformed cells, these checkpoints are defective. Cell cycle checkpoints do not operate during the early cleavage divisions of invertebrates and lower vertebrates and it has recently been suggested that the same may be true of the early human embryo[30].

CONCLUSIONS

The impact that the arrest of one or more blastomeres during cleavage will have on pre- and postimplantation development depends on the stage at which the arrest occurs, and what proportion of the embryo is effectively eliminated from partaking in development. Results from animal studies have shown clearly that even a single surviving blastomere at the 2-cell stage, where half the embryonic mass has been lost, can give rise to live young[31–33]. However, if the embryonic mass is reduced still further, implantation is compromised. Rossant[34], for example, has shown that isolated 4-cell blastomeres in the mouse can implant, but only a minority develop after implantation, whereas isolated 8-cell blastomeres rarely implant.

In the human, there is increasing evidence that embryos with a reduced cellular mass are capable of implantation and normal development. The first pregnancy to be reported for a cryopreserved embryo resulted from transfer of an embryo in which only five out of the eight blastomeres had remained intact after thawing[35]. More recently, the advent of pre-implantation genetic diagnosis for couples who are at risk of transmitting an inherited defect has provided direct evidence. The pre-implantation development of 8-cell embryos from which one or two cells have been removed is not adversely affected[36], and following identification and transfer of unaffected embryos, healthy babies have now been born[37]. This suggests that the arrest of one or two cells at the 8-cell stage (or the equivalent at other stages) should not have a significant effect on pre- or postimplantation development. However, it is clear that the redundancy of a larger proportion of the cells of an embryo, particularly during early cleavage, could have a negative impact on later implantation and development.

REFERENCES

1. Human Fertilisation and Embryo Authority (HFEA) (1994). *Annual Report*. (London: HFEA)
2. Hardy, K. (1993). Development of human blastocysts *in vitro*. In Bavister, B. (ed.) *Preimplantation Embryo Development*, pp.184–99. (New York: Springer-Verlag)
3. Telford, N.A., Watson, A.J. and Schultz, G.A. (1990). Transition from maternal to embryonic control in early mammalian development: a comparison of several species. *Mol. Reprod. Dev.*, **26**, 90–100
4. Bolton, V.N., Hawes, S.M., Taylor, C.T. and Parsons, J.H. (1989). Development of spare human preimplantation embryos *in vitro*: an analysis of the correlations among gross morphology, cleavage rates, and development to the blastocyst. *J. IVF and Embryo Transfer*, **6**, 30–5
5. Watson, A.J., Hogan, A., Hahnel, A. and Schultz, G.A. (1993). Activation of the embryonic genome: comparison between mouse and bovine development. In Bavister, B.D. (ed.) *Preimplantation Embryo Development*, pp. 115–30. (New York: Springer-Verlag)
6. Tesarik, J., Kopecny, V., Plachot, M. and Mandelbaum, J. (1986). Activation of nucleolar and extranucleolar RNA synthesis and changes in the ribosomal content of human embryos developing *in vitro*. *J. Reprod. Fertil.*, **78**, 463–70
7. Tesarik, J., Kopecny, V., Plachot, M., Mandelbaum, J., Da Lage, C. and Flechon, J.E. (1986). Nucleologenesis in the human embryo developing *in vitro*: ultrastructural and autoradiographic analysis. *Dev. Biol.*, **115**, 193–203
8. Braude, P.R., Bolton, V. and Moore, S. (1988). Human gene expression first occurs between the four- and eight-cell stages of preimplantation development. *Nature (London)* **332**, 459–61
9. Chatot, C.L., Ziomek, C.A., Bavister, B.D., Lewis, J.L. and Torres, I. (1989). An improved culture medium supports development of random-bred 1-cell mouse embryos *in vitro*. *J. Reprod. Fertil.*, **86**, 679–88
10. Brown, J.J. and Whittingham, D.G. (1992). The dynamic provision of different energy substrates improves development of one-cell random-bred mouse embryos *in vitro*. *J. Reprod. Fertil.*, **95**, 503–11
11. Schini, S.A. and Bavister, B.D. (1988). Two-cell block to development of cultured hamster embryos is caused by phosphate and glucose. *Biol. Reprod.*, **39**, 1183–92
12. Reed, M.L., Jin, D.I. and Petters, R.M. (1992). Glucose and inorganic phosphate inhibits rat 8-cell embryo development. *Theriogenology*, **37**, 282
13. Thompson, J.G., Simpson, A.C., Pugh, P.A. and Tervit, H.R. (1992).

Requirement for glucose during *in vitro* culture of sheep preimplantation embryos. *Mol. Reprod. Dev.*, **31**, 253–7

14. Seshagiri, P.B. and Bavister, B.D. (1989). Phosphate is required for inhibition by glucose of development of hamster 8-cell embryos *in vitro*. *Biol. Reprod.*, **40**, 607–14

15. Seshagiri, P.B. and Bavister, B.D. (1989). Glucose inhibits development of hamster 8-cell embryos *in vitro*. *Biol. Reprod.*, **40**, 599–606

16. Conaghan, J., Handyside, A.H., Winston, R.M.L. and Leese, H.J. (1993). Effects of pyruvate and glucose on the development of human preimplantation embryos *in vitro*. *J. Reprod. Fertil.*, **99**, 87–95

17. Bavister, B.D. and McKiernan, S.H. (1993). Regulation of hamster embryo development *in vitro* by amino acids. In Bavister, B.D. (ed.) *Preimplantation Embryo Development*, pp. 57–72. (New York: Springer-Verlag)

18. Schultz, G.A., Kaye, P.L., McKay, D.J. and Johnson, M.H. (1981). Endogenous amino acid pool sizes in mouse eggs and preimplantation embryos. *J. Reprod. Fertil.*, **61**, 387–93

19. Nasr Esfahani, M., Johnson, M.H. and Aitken, R.J. (1990). The effect of iron and iron chelators on the *in-vitro* block to development of the mouse preimplantation embryo: BAT6 a new medium for improved culture of mouse embryos *in vitro*. *Hum. Reprod.*, **5**, 997–1003

20. Nasr Esfahani, M.H. and Johnson, M.H. (1992). Quantitative analysis of cellular glutathione in early preimplantation mouse embryos developing *in vivo* and *in vitro*. *Hum. Reprod.*, **7**, 1281–90

21. Nasr Esfahani, M.H. and Johnson, M.H. (1992). How does transferrin overcome the *in vitro* block to development of the mouse preimplantation embryo? *J. Reprod. Fertil.*, **96**, 41–8

22. Nasr Esfahani, M.H., Winston, N.J. and Johnson, M.H. (1992). Effects of glucose, glutamine, ethylenediaminetetraacetic acid and oxygen tension on the concentration of reactive oxygen species and on development of the mouse preimplantation embryo *in vitro*. *J. Reprod. Fertil.*, **96**, 219–31

23. Gardner, D.K. and Lane, M. (1993). Amino acids and ammonium regulate mouse embryo development in culture. *Biol. Reprod.*, **48**, 377–85

24. Winston, N.J., Braude, P.R., Pickering, S.J., George, M.A., Cant, A., Currie, J. and Johnson, M.H. (1991). The incidence of abnormal morphology and nucleocytoplasmic ratios in 2-, 3- and 5-day human pre-embryos. *Hum. Reprod.*, **6**, 17–24

25. Hardy, K., Winston, R.M.L. and Handyside, A.H. (1993). Binucleate cells in human preimplantation embryos *in vitro*: failure of cytokinesis during cleavage. *J. Reprod. Fertil.*, **98**, 549–58

26. Munné, S., Lee, A., Rosenwaks, Z., Grifo, J. and Cohen, J. (1993).

Diagnosis of major chromosome aneuploidies in human preimplantation embryos. *Hum. Reprod.*, **8**, 2185–91

27. Harper, J.C., Coonen, E., Handyside, A.H., Winston, R.M.L., Hopman, A. and Delhanty, J.D.A. (1995). Mosaicism of autosomes and sex chromosomes in morphologically normal, monospermic preimplantation human embryos. *Prenat. Diagn.*, **15**, 41–9

28. Hartwell, L.H. and Weinert, T.A. (1989). Checkpoints: controls that ensure the order of cell cycle events. *Science*, **246**, 629–34

29. Murray, A.W. (1992). Creative blocks: cell-cycle checkpoints and feedback controls. *Nature (London)*, **359**, 599–604

30. Delhanty, J.D.A. and Handyside, A.H. (1995). The origin of genetic defects in the human and their detection in the pre-implantation embryo. In Charlton, H.C. (ed.) *Oxford Reviews of Reproductive Biology*, vol. 17. (Oxford: Oxford University Press) in press

31. Tarkowski, A.K. (1959). Experimental studies on regulation in the development of isolated blastomeres of mouse eggs. *Acta Theriologica*, **3**, 191–267

32. Tarkowski, A.K. (1959). Experiments on the development of isolated blastomeres of mouse eggs. *Nature (London)*, **184**, 1286–7

33. Papaioannou, V.E., Mkandawire, J. and Biggers, J.D. (1989). Development and phenotypic variability of genetically identical half mouse embryos. *Development*, **106**, 817–27

34. Rossant, J. (1976). Postimplantation development of blastomeres isolated from 4 and 8-cell mouse eggs. *J. Embryol. Exp. Morph.*, **36**, 283–90

35. Trounson, A.O. and Mohr, L. (1983). Human pregnancy following cryopreservation, thawing and transfer of an eight-cell embryo. *Nature (London)*, **305**, 707

36. Hardy, K., Martin, K.L., Leese, H.J., Winston, R.M. and Handyside, A.H. (1990). Human preimplantation development *in vitro* is not adversely affected by biopsy at the 8-cell stage. *Hum. Reprod.*, **5**, 708–14

37. Harper, J. and Handyside, A.H. (1994). The current status of preimplantation diagnosis. *Curr. Obs. Gynaecol.*, **4**, 143–9

2

Assessment of embryo nutritional requirements and role of co-culture techniques

H. J. Leese, M. Alexiou, M. T. Comer, V. K. Lamb and J. G. Thompson

INTRODUCTION

The experimental approaches used to assess the nutritional requirements of pre-implantation mammalian embryos have changed little since the pioneering work in the 1960s, notably by Biggers, Brinster, Wales, Whitten and Whittingham, which led to the discovery of media which could sustain the development of mouse zygotes into blastocysts in culture. Although modern approaches are technically more sophisticated, they still fall into four types, similar to those which were used 25–30 years ago; the aims of which are:

(1)   To examine the effect on development of modifying embryo culture media.

(2)   To measure the uptake of nutrients at different stages of development.

(3)   To determine the concentration of nutrients in the lumen of the female reproductive tract.

(4)   To grow pre-implantation embryos in association with somatic cells in co-culture, in order to elucidate the advantage to development (if any) conferred.

These four approaches are considered in turn, below.

11

EMBRYO CULTURE MEDIA

Work in the 1960s showed that early mouse embryos would develop in relatively simple media containing mineral salts, a macromolecule such as albumin and one or more energy sources – typically, pyruvate, which is obligatory for the first cleavage division, lactate and glucose, which, as sole substrate, will support development from the 4–8-cell stage[1]. Amino acids are not required until the onset of true growth, at blastocyst expansion and hatching. Numerous variations on this theme have been devised and used to culture the pre-implantation embryos of many species. There are perhaps three recent findings of most interest. Firstly, the realization that different media can sustain equivalent development[2], suggesting that embryos can, to some extent, adapt to their environment. Such adaptation enables them to survive in the female tract, where the environment will be changing constantly. Secondly, it was found that plasma-level concentrations of glucose are inhibitory to early development of embryos in a variety of species[3–7]. This most probably relates to the relatively low levels of glucose found in oviduct fluid (see below) and the low capacity for glucose utilization during the early cleavage stages[8,9]. A third finding was that the addition of mixed amino acids is highly beneficial only when ammonium ions, produced from amino acid metabolism and degradation, are removed from the culture system[10,11]. The accumulation of NH_4^+ ions that occurs when culturing embryos is a good example of a toxin introduced into culture, and therefore an artefact of the *in vitro* system. *In situ*, embryos would not be exposed to high levels of this and other environmental toxins, since oviduct fluid is formed continuously and, at least in the sheep, normally flows out of the fimbriated end of the tube into the peritoneal cavity, following the path of least resistance[12].

NUTRIENT UPTAKE MEASUREMENTS

Early studies on the uptake of nutrients by early mammalian embryos were carried out mainly by Brinster, Wales and Whittingham, using radiolabelled substrates. They confirmed that the nutrients added to embryo culture media were, indeed, consumed by the embryos; that this metabolic activity increased sharply during the later stages of pre-implantation development[13,14]; and that blastocyst formation coincided

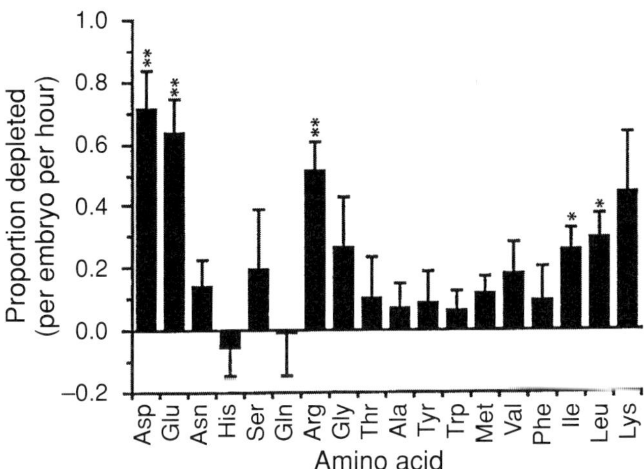

Figure 1 Mean proportional amino acid depletion rates (per embryo per hour) by groups of mouse blastocysts on day 4 of development incubated in medium containing 20 amino acids each at a concentration of 0.1 mmol/l *p < 0.05, **p < 0.01 compared with zero depletion. (From ref. 21, with permission from the *Journal of Reproduction and Fertility*)

with a pronounced rise in glucose consumption. These findings have been confirmed using a non-invasive approach which obviates the use of radiolabelled substrates[15–18] and can be used safely with single human embryos that are replaced in the uterus[19]. Moreover, the rise in glucose uptake during the later stages has emerged as a universal phenomenon amongst all the species studied[8,9].

A considerable body of literature exists on the uptake of single amino acids by pre-implantation embryos, largely from studies on the mouse, where competition experiments have been used to identify a range of transport systems, as well as their pattern of expression throughout development[20]. We have recently re-examined the question of amino-acid uptake by pre-implantation embryos by applying the non-invasive approach to groups of about 30 mouse blastocysts, 4 and 5 days after human chorionic gonadotrophin (hCG) treatment. Since early embryos are exposed to the full range of amino acids in the female tract, we have measured the simultaneous depletion of 18 out of a mixture of 20 amino acids using high performance liquid chromatography[21]. The mouse blastocysts depleted the medium of amino acids at widely differing rates; the key amino acids sought by embryos on both days 4 and 5 being aspartate, glutamate, arginine, isoleucine and leucine (Figure 1). Curiously, glutamine, which has attracted a good deal of interest, and is frequently added to embryo culture media, was not depleted from the medium at a significant rate on either day. Data such as these may require us to reconsider the addition of single amino acids to embryo culture media.

NUTRIENT COMPOSITION OF THE FEMALE REPRODUCTIVE TRACT

Holmdahl and Mastroianni[22] cannulated rabbit oviducts *in situ*, and showed that the oviduct fluid collected contained pyruvate, glucose and lactate. We have measured the glucose, pyruvate and lactate content of hydrosalpinx fluid[23], of three samples of neat human tubal fluid[24], and of fluid formed during the vascular perfusion of isolated human tubes removed at hysterectomy[25]. The most striking finding from all these studies is the low concentration of glucose in the human tubal lumen which, at about 0.5 mmol/l, is approximately 10 times below that routinely used in embryo culture (5.5 mmol/l), and studies in other species have similarly reported glucose concentrations significantly lower than in plasma[26,27]. These findings provide some physiological justification for omitting or lowering the glucose concentration in embryo culture media, at least during the early stages. When this was done in spare human embryos, blastocyst development and cell number were enhanced[28].

CO-CULTURE

Pioneering experiments in this field were carried out by Whittingham, Biggers and Gwatkin in the late 1960s. It was shown that mouse embryos, whose development was normally blocked at the 2-cell stage in culture, would resume development if placed in isolated Fallopian tubes maintained as whole organ cultures[29]. Current interest in exploiting the potential of the tube to facilitate embryo development stems from the work of Gandolfi and Moor[30] who reported that sheep embryo development in a 'complex' medium (M199) supplemented with serum was superior if oviduct cells from the flushings of the tract were included.

The major problem in this field is the need to reconcile the different nutrient requirements of the embryo and supporting somatic cells. Early mammalian embryos are undifferentiated, largely autonomous structures which can develop in relatively simple media in culture, whereas somatic cells are highly differentiated, dependent *in situ* on interactions with other cell types, and require complex media for their maintenance. Moreover, the phenotype of the supporting layer of somatic cells in culture has not been characterized in sufficient detail. For example, the phenotype of established cell lines (e.g. Vero, BRL), which have been used widely in co-culture studies, is well-characterized. However, when cells from the female tract have been used in co-culture experiments, notably from the oviduct, it has generally been assumed that their *in vitro* phenotype is similar to that exhibited *in situ* – an assumption which is not justified. The oviduct epithelium, *in situ*, is comprised of asymmetric, polarized, ciliated and non-ciliated cells[31] supported by an underlying stroma, through which hormonal sensitivity may be mediated[32,33]. In most of the oviduct preparations used for co-culture, little attention has been paid to cell polarity, the maintenance of cilia, the expression of epithelial cell type markers, or the role of the stroma. Thus, it is not surprising that controversy exists over the nature of any advantage conferred by embryo–oviduct co-culture[34,35]; there is insufficient knowledge of the extent to which the phenotype of oviduct cells *in vitro* reflects that exhibited *in situ*.

In an attempt to address these problems, we have isolated oviduct epithelial cells from the sheep[36], rabbit[37], human[38] and mouse[39] and grown them in primary culture on permeable cell supports, in the hope that they would form a polarized monolayer similar to that exhibited *in situ*. The results indicate different, apparently tissue-specific and media-dependent responses.

Sheep

Epithelial cells were obtained from the oviducts of sheep by gently scraping the oviduct surface and collecting the exuded cells in Medium 199. After washing, clumps of cells were plated on filter inserts coated with 2.5% poly-L-lysine and grown in Medium 199 + 10% foetal calf serum (FCS) or Medium 199 + 10% charcoal-stripped, steroid-free FCS at 39°C in 5% CO_2 in air for 6 days, by which time a confluent monolayer had developed from clumps of cells. The phenotype of cells within the

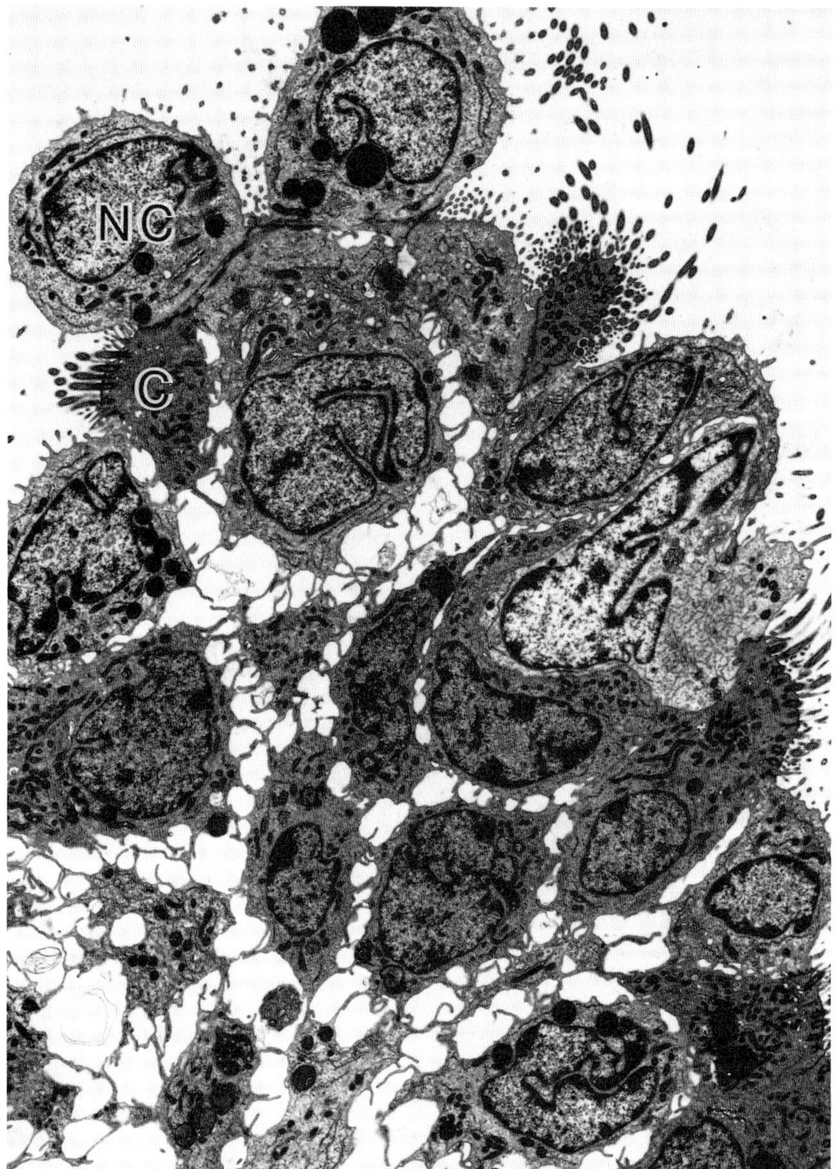

Figure 2 Clump of ovine oviduct epithelial cells cultured for 6 days in Medium 199 supplemented with foetal calf serum. Note that most cells have retained much of their *in vivo* morphology, despite the absence of a functional basement membrane (C = ciliated cell. NC = non-ciliated cell). (× 4130)

clumps and monolayer were examined by both histological analysis (using periodic acid–Schiff's (PAS) reagent), and transmission (TEM) and scanning electron microscopy (SEM). Cells within clumps retained much of the oviduct phenotype, with distinct cilia and secretory functions retained (Figure 2). Cells comprising the monolayer were harder to characterize, with some evidence of polarization (microvilli and occasionally cilia on the apical surface) but PAS staining revealed that a proportion of cells were actively synthesizing PAS-positive staining material. Under TEM, a similar proportion of cells had many characteristics of cells actively synthesizing polypeptides. The proportion of PAS-positive cells was also influenced by serum treatment and the presence of steroids. In particular, the addition of progesterone and oestradiol (together) greatly increased the proportion of monolayer cells staining positively for PAS.

Rabbit, human and mouse

We have used an enzymic digestion method originally devised to isolate epithelial cells from the mouse uterus[40,41]. Slit oviducts are incubated in a pancreatin/trypsin solution and the cells released cultured on collagen-impregnated inserts in a mixture of Ham's F12 and Dulbecco's modified Eagle's medium supplemented with foetal calf serum, Nu-serum and glutamine. Rabbit oviduct cells grown under these conditions form a confluent, polarized monolayer, as demonstrated by immunocytochemistry, electron microscopy and the asymmetric nature of glucose uptake and lactate output[37,42,43]. Human tubal epithelial cells behave similarly[38] although their *in situ* morphology is less well-preserved. However, in both the rabbit and human cultures, substantial numbers of cilia are lost, in contrast with the preparation used for the sheep.

The mouse oviduct posed considerable problems; cells cultured in the medium which successfully supported rabbit and human oviduct growth assumed confluence in 3–5 days, but grew as multiple layers (Figure 3) and failed to show asymmetric glucose uptake and lactate output.

With regard to co-culture and in an attempt to mimic the *in vivo* situation, one-cell mouse zygotes were placed in medium M16 (i.e. a simple, serum-free, defined medium, likely to reflect better the composition of oviduct fluid) on the upper, apical surface of the oviduct

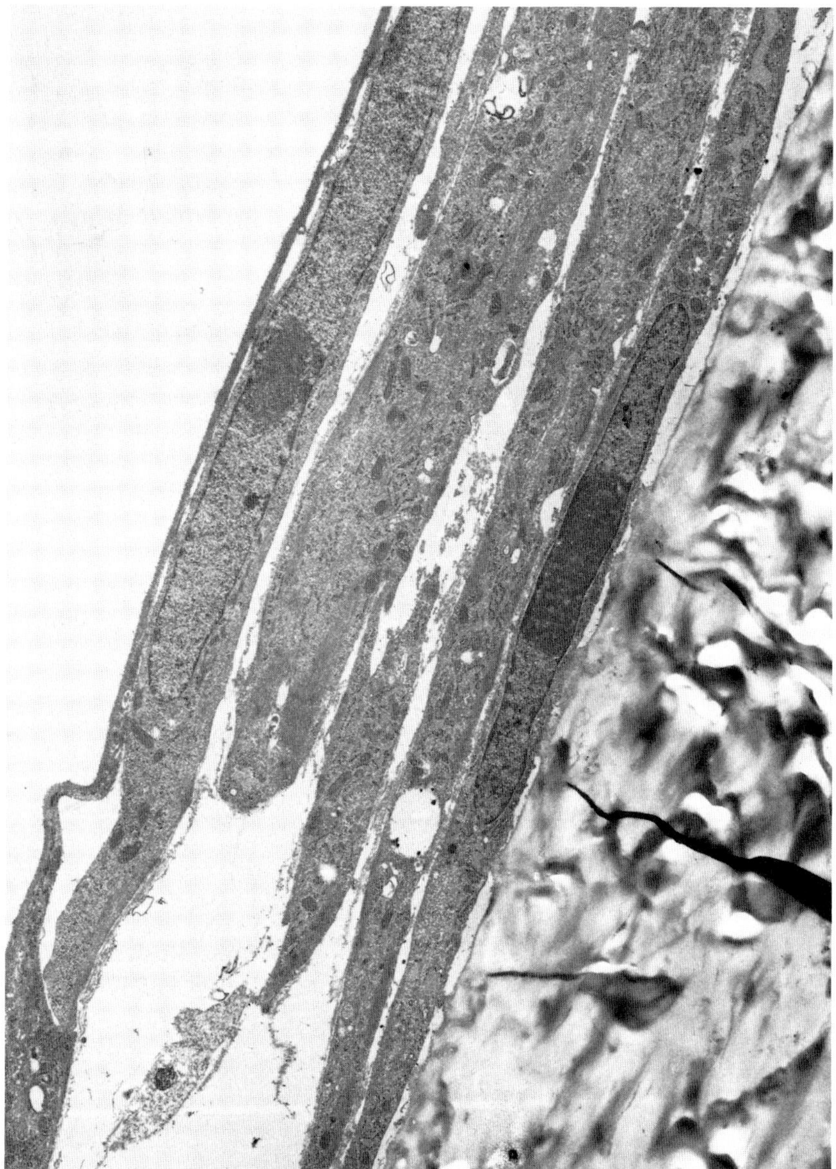

Figure 3 Mouse oviduct epithelial cells isolated by enzyme digestion and grown on a collagen-impregnated filter in Ham's F12 and Dulbecco's modified Eagle's medium supplemented with foetal calf serum, Nu-serum and glutamine. Note multiple layers and elongated cells. (× 2895)

cells, with the basal surface, beneath the collagen filters, bathed in the more complex cell culture media. However, no convincing, positive effect of co-culture could be demonstrated.

CONCLUSIONS ON THE EFFICACY OF PRE-IMPLANTATION EMBRYO/SOMATIC CELL CO-CULTURE

Development of embryos from a wide range of mammalian species, particularly the later stages of pre-implantation development, are assisted by the presence of somatic cells under certain conditions. However, no convincing advantage of the use of oviduct, as opposed to other cell types, has been shown. However, the phenotype of oviduct cells *in situ* and *in vitro* has not been sufficiently characterized and until this has been done, there is no justification for concluding that the oviduct cells used for co-culture are truly 'oviductal'.

THE FUTURE

As indicated earlier in this review, pre-implantation embryos within the oviduct are exposed to a variety of environments, as detailed by Leese[44]. As our understanding of the dynamic nature of the environment within the oviduct lumen continues to emerge, embryo culture will attempt to reflect these changes, but it is unlikely that static systems will be appropriate. In contrast, perfusion culture systems may enable developing embryos to be exposed to gradients of energy substrates, growth factors, gas tension and ionic composition, while continuously removing potential metabolic toxins[45]. Indeed, an early prototype perfusion system supported the development of *in vitro*-produced bovine embryos to the blastocyst stage, albeit at lower than acceptable levels (J.G. Thompson, unpublished data).

ACKNOWLEDGEMENTS

I IJL thanks The Wellcome Trust and The Medical Research Council for financial support.

REFERENCES

1. Biggers, J.D., Whitten, W.K. and Whittingham, D.G. (1971). The culture of mouse embryo *in vitro*. In Daniel, J.C. (ed.) *Methods of Mammalian Embryology* pp. 7–21. (San Francisco: Freeman)
2. Lawitts, J.A. and Biggers, J.D. (1991). Optimization of mouse embryo culture media using simplex methods. *J. Reprod. Fertil.*, **91**, 543–56
3. Schini, S.A. and Bavister, B.D. (1988). Two cell block to development of cultured hamster embryos is caused by phosphate and glucose. *Biol. Reprod.*, **39**, 1183–92
4. Chatot, C.L., Ziomek, C.A., Bavister, B.D., Lewis, J.L. and Torres, I. (1989). An improved culture medium supports development of random-bred 1-cell mouse embryos *in vitro*. *J. Reprod. Fertil.*, **86**, 679–88
5. Thompson, J.G., Simpson, A.C., Pugh, P.A. and Tervit, H.R. (1992). Requirement for glucose during *in vitro* culture of sheep preimplantation embryos. *Mol. Reprod. Dev.*, **31**, 253–7
6. Matsuyama, K., Miyakoshi, H. and Fukui, Y. (1993). Effect of glucose levels during the *in vitro* culture in synthetic oviduct fluid medium on *in vitro* development of bovine oocytes matured and fertilized *in vitro*. *Theriogenology*, **40**, 596–605
7. Conaghan, J., Handyside, A.H., Winston, R.M.L. and Leese, H.J. (1993). Effects of pyruvate and glucose on the development of human preimplantation embryos *in vitro*. *J. Reprod. Fertil.*, **99**, 87–95
8. Leese, H.J. (1991). Metabolism of the preimplantation mammalian embryo. In Milligan, S. R. (ed.) *Oxford Rev. Reprod. Biol.*, **13**, 35–72
9. Rieger, D. (1992). Relationships between energy metabolism and development of early mammalian embryos. *Theriogenology*, **37**, 75–93
10. Gardner, D.K. and Lane, M. (1993). Amino acids and ammonium regulate mouse embryo development in culture. *Biol. Reprod.*, **48**, 377–85
11. Gardner, D.K., Lane, M., Spitzer, A. and Batt, P.A. (1994). Enhanced rates of cleavage and development of sheep zygotes cultured to the blastocyst stage *in vitro* in the absence of serum and somatic cells: amino acids, vitamins, and culturing embryos in groups stimulate development. *Biol. Reprod.*, **50**, 390–400
12. Bellvé, A.R. and MacDonald, M.F. (1968). Directional flow of Fallopian tube secretion in the Romney ewe. *J. Reprod. Fertil.*, **15**, 357–64
13. Brinster, R.L., (1973). Nutrition and metabolism of the ovum, zygote and blastocyst. In Greep, R.O. and Astwood, E.B. (eds.) *Handbook of Physiology*, Vol. II, pp. 165–85. (Washington D.C.: American Physiological Society)
14. Wales, R.G. (1975). Maturation of the mammalian embryo: biochemical aspects. *Biol. Reprod.*, **12**, 66–81

15. Leese, H.J. and Barton, A.M. (1984). Pyruvate and glucose uptake by mouse ova and preimplantation embryos. *J. Reprod. Fertil.*, **72**, 9–13

16. Leese, H.J. (1987). Analysis of embryos by non-invasive methods. *Hum. Reprod.*, **2**, 37–40

17. Gardner, D.K. and Leese, H.J. (1987). Assessment of embryo viability prior to transfer by the non-invasive measurement of glucose uptake. *J. Exp. Zool.*, **242**, 103–5

18. Gardner, D.K. and Leese, H.J. (1993). Assessment of embryo metabolism and viability. In Trounson, A. and Gardner, D.K. (eds.) *Handbook of In Vitro Fertilization*, pp. 195–211. (Boca Raton, Florida, USA: CRC Press)

19. Conaghan, J., Hardy, K., Handyside, A.H., Winston, R.M.L. and Leese, H.J. (1993). Selection criteria for human embryo transfer: a comparison of pyruvate uptake and morphology. *J. Assist. Reprod. Genet.*, **10**, 21–30

20. Van Winkle, L.J. (1988). Amino acid transport in developing animal oocytes and early conceptuses. *Biochim. Biophys. Acta*, **947**, 173–208

21. Lamb, V.K. and Leese, H.J. (1994). Uptake of a mixture of amino acids by mouse blastocysts. *J. Reprod. Fertil.*, **102**, 169–75

22. Holmdahl, T.H. and Mastroianni, L. Jr (1965). Continuous collection of rabbit oviduct secretions at low temperature. *Fertil. Steril.*, **16**, 587–95

23. Gott, A.L., Hardy, K., Winston, R.M.L. and Leese, H.J. (1990). The nutrition and environment of the early human embryo. *Proc. Nutr. Soc.*, **49**, 2A

24. Leese, H.J. and Dickens, C.J. (1992). Tubal physiology and function. In Templeton, A.A. and Drife, J.O. (eds.) *Infertility*, pp. 157–68. (London: Springer Verlag)

25. Dickens, C.J., Maguiness, S.D., Comer, M.T., Palmer, A., Rutherford, A.J. and Leese, H.J. (1995). Human tubal fluid: formation and composition during vascular perfusion of the human Fallopian tube. *Human Reprod.*, in press

26. Gardner, D.K. and Leese, H.J. (1990). Concentrations of nutrients in mouse oviduct fluid and their effects on embryo development and metabolism *in vitro. Reprod. Fertil.*, **88**, 361–8

27. Nichol, R., Hunter, R.H.F., Gardner, D.K., Leese, H.J. and Cooke, G.M. (1992). Concentrations of energy substrates in oviductal fluid and blood plasma of pigs during the periovulatory period. *J. Reprod. Fertil.*, **96**, 699–707

28. Conaghan, J., Handyside, A.H., Winston, R.M.L. and Leese, H.J. (1993). Effects of pyruvate and glucose on the development of human preimplantation embryos *in vitro. J. Reprod. Fertil.*, **99**, 87–95

29. Whittingham, D.G. and Biggers, J.D. (1967). Fallopian tube and early cleavage in the mouse. *Nature (London)*, **213**, 942–3

30. Gandolfi, F. and Moor, R.M. (1987). Stimulation of early embryonic development in the sheep by co-culture with oviduct epithelial cells. *J. Reprod. Fertil.*, **81**, 23–8

31. Leese, H.J. (1988). The formation and function of oviduct fluid. *J. Reprod. Fertil.*, **82**, 843–56

32. Brenner, R.M., West, N.B. and McClellan, M.C. (1990). Estrogen and progestin receptors in the reproductive tract of male and female primates. *Biol. Reprod.*, **42**, 11–19

33. Amso, N.N., Crow, J. and Shaw, R.W. (1994). Comparative immunohisto-chemical study of oestrogen and progesterone receptors in the Fallopian tube and uterus at different stages of the menstrual cycle and the meno-pause. *Hum. Reprod.*, **9**, 1027–37

34. Bongso, A., Fong, C.-Y., Ng, S.-C. and Ratnam, S. (1993). The search for improved *in–vitro* systems should not be ignored: embryo co-culture may be one of them. *Hum. Reprod.*, **8**, 1155–60

35. Bavister, B.D. (1993). Response to the use of co-culture for embryo development. *Hum. Reprod.*, **8**, 1160–2

36. Simpson, A.C., Nixon, A.J. and Thompson, J.G. (1991). Ovine oviductal cell monolayers: effects of sera and steroids on cell populations. *Proc. Aust. Soc. Reprod. Biol.*, **23**, 99

37. Dickens, C.J., Southgate, J. and Leese, H.J. (1993). The use of cultures of rabbit oviduct epithelial cells to study the ionic basis of tubal fluid formation. *J. Reprod.Fertil.*, **98**, 603–10

38. Dickens, C.J., Skiera, L., Southgate, J. and Leese, H.J. (1993). Polarised human fallopian tubal epithelial cells in culture: a preliminary study. *Hum. Reprod.*, **8** (Suppl. 1), 57

39. Alexiou, M., Lindsay, M.T. and Leese, H.J. (1993). Co–culture of mouse oviduct epithelial cells with mouse embryos: effects of different culture media. *Hum. Reprod.*, **8** (Suppl. 1), 46–7

40. Glasser, S.R., Julian, J., Decker, G.L., Tang, J.P. and Carson D.D. (1988). Development of morphological and functional polarity in primary cultures of immature rat uterine epithelial cells. *J. Cell Biol.*, **107**, 2409–23

41. Kimber, S.J., Waterhouse, R. and Lindenberg, S. (1993). *In vitro* models for implantation in the mammalian embryo. In Bavister, B. (ed.) *Preimplantation Embryo Development, Serono Symposia USA,* pp. 244–63. (New York: Springer–Verlag)

42. Edwards, L.J. and Leese, H.J. (1993). Glucose transport and metabolism in rabbit oviduct epithelial cells. *J. Reprod. Fertil.*, **99**, 585–91

43. Leese, H.J., Brewis, I.A., Edwards, L.J., Gray, S.M., Skiera, L.S. and Winston, R.M.L. (1994). Biochemistry of tubal secretions. In Grudzinskas, J.G., Chapman, M.G., Chard, T. and Djahanbakhch, O. (eds.) *The Fallopian*

Tube, Clinical and Surgical Aspects, pp. 53–62. (London: Springer–Verlag)
44.   Leese, H.J. (1990). Environment of the preimplantation embryo. In Edwards, R.G. (ed.) *Establishing a Successful Human Pregnancy*, pp. 143–54 (New York: Raven Press)
45.   Thompson, J.G. (1994) How well do we culture domestic ruminant embryos? Presented at the *Proceedings of the New Zealand Embryo Transfer Workshop*, Hamilton, New Zealand, January

3

Evaluation of embryo quality: the role of human cumulus and corona cells in implantation and early pregnancy

L. Gregory

INTRODUCTION

Advances in assisted reproduction techniques have made significant contributions to the understanding of the conditions necessary for oocyte maturation, fertilization and pre-embryo development, but events at the foeto-maternal interface at implantation have yet to be determined. Implantation is known to be dependant upon the interaction of a number of embryonic and maternal signals. Because of the difficulty of obtaining human material from the peri-implantation period, evidence for the process is indirect, based on changes in maternal physiology in advance of implantation or during the peri-implantation period[1,2]. These changes distinguish between conception and non-conception cycles but are a reflection of implantation and do not necessarily provide the impetus for the process.

It is accepted that implantation will require a viable embryo, receptive endometrium and, because of the semi-allogenic nature of the foetus, immunosuppression. Where implantation occurs, then all three parameters must be favourable. However, endometrial receptivity is clearly not a factor in those *in vitro* fertilization (IVF) cycles where some embryos implant while other embryos from the same cohort fail.

Much research has been directed at improving outcome from IVF and identifying those aspects of the treatment (particularly pre-embryo

Table 1 11β-hydroxysteroid dehydrogenase activity (11β-HSD) in cultured granulosa–lutein cells and outcome from *in vitro* fertilization–embryo transfer. (After Michael and colleagues[29])

	Clinical pregnancies (%)	Not pregnant (%)
Results for series (*n* = 79)	34.2	65.8
11β-HSD-positive cells (*n* = 39)	0	100
11β-HSD-negative cells (*n* = 40)	67.5★	32.5

★Pregnancies per embryo transfer: 73%

quality) which contribute to implantation. The parameters which are most commonly used in the assessment of embryo quality are morphology and cleavage rates[3,4]. However, embryos which fall into the best categories for these parameters frequently fail to implant. Embryo quality has also been evaluated by assay of supernatant from embryo culture. This has allowed the identification of systems which promote implantation[5,6]. Whilst the use of these systems may increase the probability of pregnancy, they fail to distinguish between those embryos which fail to implant and those which will result in pregnancy.

The scale of embryo loss may be calculated from the latest UK data which demonstrate that approximately 90% of embryos selected for transfer fail to implant[7]. Whilst it is postulated that between 30 and 60% of embryo loss is the result of chromosome anomaly[8,9] the remaining loss of apparently viable embryos is unexplained.

Two aspects of ovarian cell function have recently been identified which have the potential to provide a predictor of failed implantation from IVF–embryo transfer (IVF–ET). Thus, Michael and colleagues[10] identified a link between the expression of 11β-hydroxysteroid dehydrogenase (11β-HSD) by cultured granulosa cells and failed implantation from IVF–ET (Table 1); no pregnancies resulted from cycles where cultured granulosa lutein cells expressed 11β-HSD, whereas the pregnancy rate was 73% from cycles where granulosa cells did not express 11β-HSD

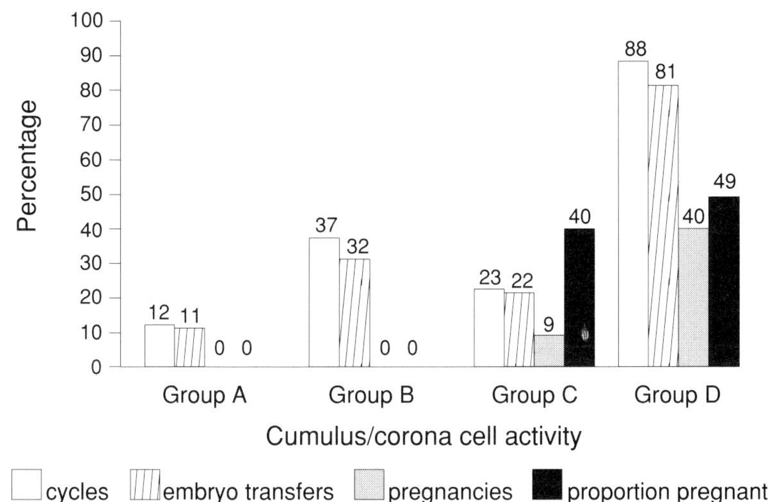

Figure 1 Cumulus and corona cell proliferation *in vitro* and pregnancy from *in vitro* fertilization–embryo transfer. Where Group A exhibited no activity *in vitro*, Group B exhibited minimal transformation and no proliferative activity, Group C exhibited varied proliferative activity and Group D exhibited extensive proliferation. (After Gregory and co-workers[11])

in culture. Similarly, Gregory and co-workers[11] demonstrated a correlation between the failure of cumulus and corona cells to proliferate *in vitro* and failure of implantation from IVF–ET (Figure 1).

Thus, two aspects of ovarian cell function have been identified which have the potential to predict the failure of implantation from IVF–ET, without influencing fertilization or cleavage rates and, therefore, provide a means of evaluating embryo quality. However, evidence now indicates that the cumulus/corona complex, in addition to providing a marker of embryo quality, has the potential to influence the peri-implantation processes and early pregnancy.

OBSERVATIONS ON CULTURED CUMULUS AND CORONA CELLS

Morphology

The cumulus comprises relatively large, spherical cells approximately 18 μm in diameter that characteristically include numerous refractile

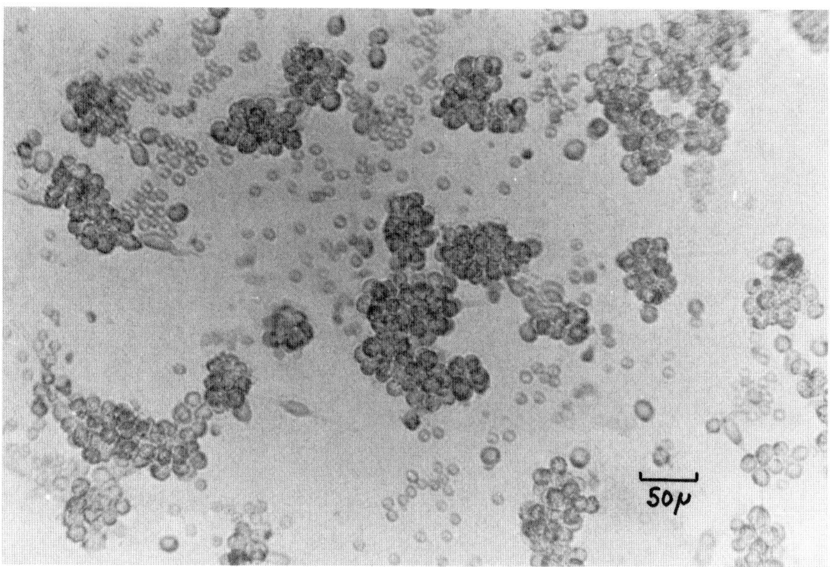

Figure 2 Cumulus cells exhibiting a characteristic spherical form. (Unstained cells photographed under liquid paraffin; bright field illumination)

intracytoplasmic granules (Figure 2). The cumulus mass invests the intra-follicular oocyte and undergoes morphological change, namely expansion and mucification as the oocyte matures, so that the cells increasingly become embedded in a mucoid matrix. These morphological changes occur in response to both endogenous and exogenous factors – e.g. luteinizing hormone (LH) and human chorionic gonadotrophin (hCG) respectively. The mature oocyte is invested by an expanded cumulus mass, with the innermost cells (the corona radiata) remaining as a dense, discrete layer adjacent to the zona pellucida. Following both *in vitro* and *in vivo* insemination, the cumulus is dispersed by the action of spermatozoa but the corona is retained by the fertilized oocyte. Most IVF programmes, however, incorporate a check for fertilization which involves the mechanical removal of at least part of the corona.

These observations on the proliferative potential of cumulus and corona were made on cells obtained from oocytes recovered in the course of IVF treatments and cultured in HEPES-buffered Minimum Essential Medium (MEM) with Earle's salts (Life Technologies Ltd., Paisley, UK) supplemented with 0.11 g/l sodium pyruvate (Life Technologies Ltd.,

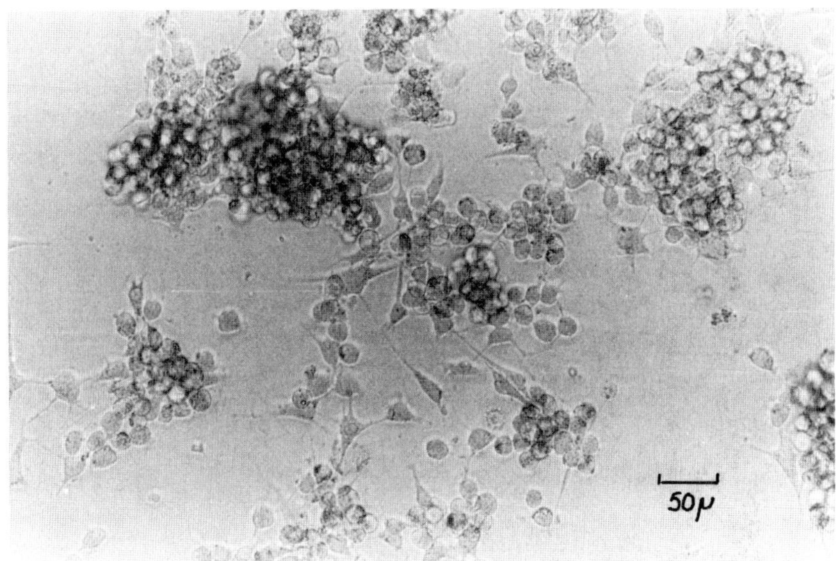

Figure 3 Transformation of cumulus cells *in vitro* in advance of proliferation. (Unstained cells photographed under liquid paraffin; bright field illumination)

Paisley, UK) and 10% (v / v) heat–inactivated patient's serum. The cultures were maintained in tissue culture treated plastic petri dishes under sterile liquid paraffin in an atmosphere of 5% CO_2 in air. Proliferative activity, exhibited by some cumulus and corona cell lines, is evident in IVF within 24 h of insemination, coincident with the check for fertilization[11]. The changes are preceded by adhesion of the cells to the culture dish and involve a transformation from the characteristic spherical appearance to a stellate form, by the extension of cytoplasmic processes (Figure 3). After 2 days culture, cumulus cells frequently form confluent monolayers up to 12 mm^2.

In systems where the cells fail to proliferate they retain their spherical appearance and form dense clumps of cells within 2–3 days of culture. Proliferation of cumulus and corona is independent of fertilization and is exhibited both by corona cells which remain adherent to the zona and those cells dispersed in the culture system at the time of the check for fertilization (Figure 4).

After several days cultured cumulus cells acquire the dense yellow staining which is usually attributed to luteinization in granulosa–lutein culture[12]. At the same time, unluteinized cells develop at the periphery of

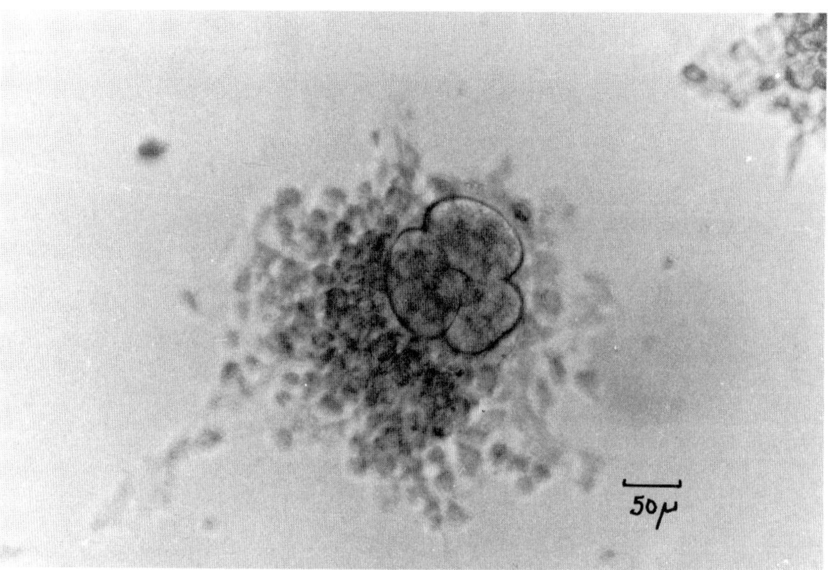

Figure 4 *In vitro* proliferative activity by corona cells retained on the zona pellucida. (Unstained cells photographed under liquid paraffin; bright field illumination)

the main cell mass and migrate in culture. These migratory cells remain unluteinized and may acquire a typically vesiculate appearance (Figure 5). Corona cells rarely show evidence of luteinization but the main cell clusters produce migratory cells which are morphologically indistinguishable from those produced in cumulus culture (author's personal observation).

Cumulus and corona cells have been maintained in culture for up to 80 days, the equivalent of 13 weeks' gestation. In such long-term cultures there is a tendency for heavily luteinized cells to become detached from the culture surface, whereas the unluteinized cells are firm in their attachment.

The significance of the potential of these cells to proliferate *in vitro* was demonstrated by the absence of pregnancies where there was a failure of cell proliferation[11] (Figure 1). Conversely, in cycles where cumulus and corona exhibited extensive proliferative activity the clinical pregnancy rate from IVF–ET was 49%. Gregory and colleagues[11] further identified a group of cycles, comprising 14% of their series, where there was variation in the proliferative capacity of these cells between oocytes of the same

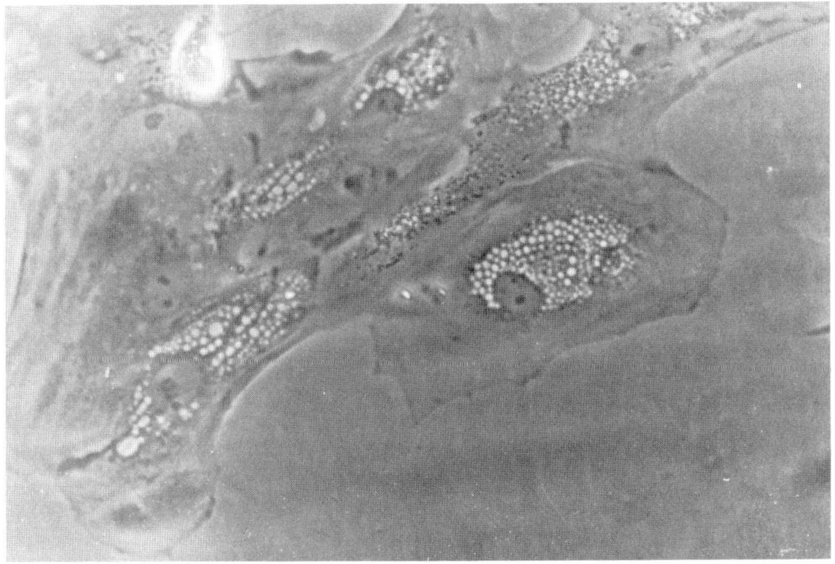

Figure 5 Migratory cells exhibiting vesiculation of the cytoplasm. (Unstained cells photographed under liquid paraffin; phase contrast illumination)

cohort – some oocytes being associated with cumulus/corona which failed to proliferate, while other oocytes were associated with cumulus/ corona exhibiting extensive proliferation (Figure 1). Embryos in the latter group were selected for transfer on the basis of their morphology in conjunction with the proliferative capacity of these cells. The pregnancy rate from IVF–ET for this group was 40%. This variation in cell potential is significant because it suggests that the phenomenon observed was an inherent feature of the cumulus complex and not a reflection of factors such as cycle management or culture techniques. Thus, a population of oocytes/embryos was identified where the failure to implant was directly related to failed proliferation of the associated cumulus/corona cells[11].

Steroidogenesis

The role of granulosa cells in steroid production is well documented. These cells are the source of 17β-oestradiol in the follicular phase and of progesterone production in the luteal phase. Granulosa–lutein cells are also the main source of steroids in early pregnancy until the placenta becomes the principal organ of steroidogenesis at 6–8 weeks' gestation[13]. Evidence has recently been produced for the role of cumulus and corona cells in steroidogenesis in the peri-implantation period and early pregnancy[14,15].

The production of 17β-oestradiol and progesterone by these cells *in vitro* was demonstrated by radioimmunoassay of culture supernatant from both cumulus and corona cells (Coat-a-Count Oestradiol and Progesterone, Diagnostic Products Ltd., Caernarfon, Gwynedd, UK) sampled daily over 14 days and stored at −4°C until required for assay.

Controls were provided by culture medium supplemented with 10% (v/v) patient's serum, as before, which had not been exposed to cells. Controls were assayed for hCG and LH (Serozyme HCG and LH, Serono Diagnostics Ltd., Wokingham, UK) in addition to 17β-oestradiol and progesterone. With the exception of hCG, all were within the negative range for their respective assays. Concentrations of hCG were marginally positive: 5–10 mIU / ml, where the negative range for the assay is < 5 mIU / ml but > 25 mIU / ml for a positive pregnancy test.

Concentrations of progesterone in cumulus culture immediately following ovulation were in the range 69–862 nmol / l per cumulus–oocyte-complex (COC) / 24 h. Progesterone levels in pooled supernatant from cumulus culture were 276–4580 nmol / l, far in excess of plasma progesterone concentrations at the same time, which were approximately 40–68 nmol / l. Progesterone concentrations *in vivo* may exceed that measured *in vitro* because the cells would be subject to the *in vivo* influences of potential stimulants such as hCG. The potential of these cells to produce high concentrations of progesterone at this time led to the hypothesis that they may make a major contribution to the priming of the endometrium[14,15].

A comparison of progesterone concentrations in pregnancy-related cumulus / corona culture with those from failed conception cycles shows that they fall within the same range. However, in non-pregnant cycles progesterone concentrations tended to decline over the 14-day period from oocyte collection, whilst in pregnancy-related cultures the progesterone concentrations remained stable (mean ± SD:234 ± 32 nmol / l; see Figure 6). This parallels the pattern seen in plasma progesterones over the same period.

Cumulus and corona cultures from conception cycles were maintained for up to 80 days. The cells continued their steroidogenic activity

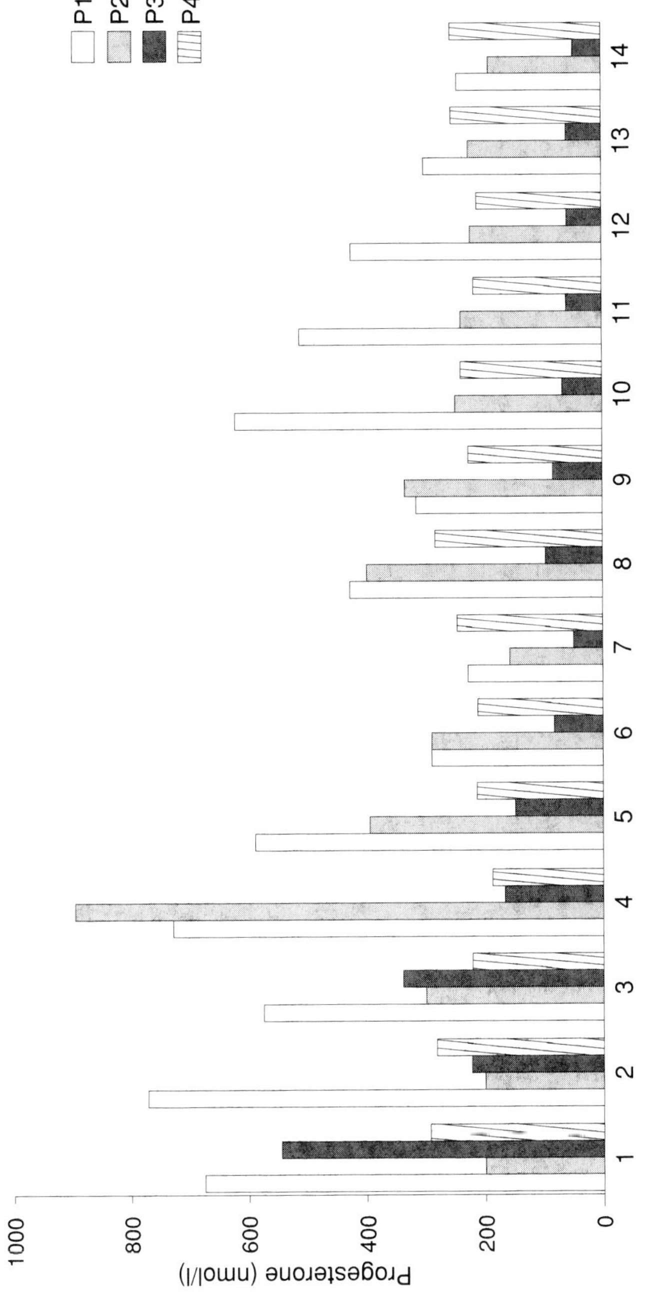

Figure 6 Progesterone concentrations in supernatant from cumulus culture (nmol/l per cumulus–oocyte complex per 24 h), where P1–P3 were associated with non-conception cycles, and cells from P4 were pregnancy-related. Controls: <1.0–2.7nmol/l

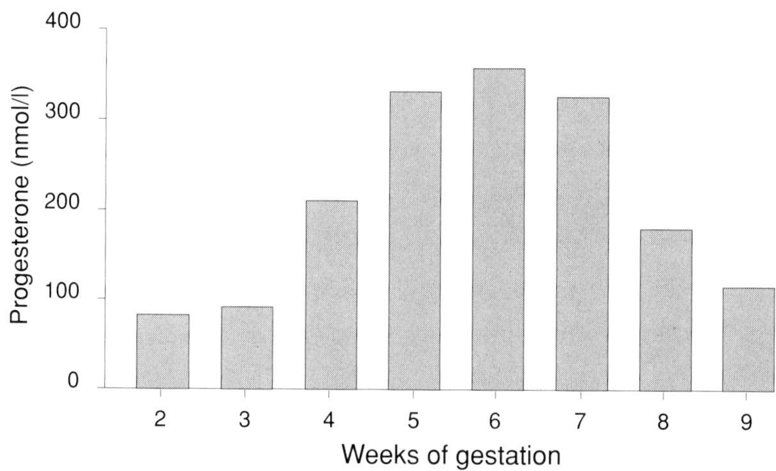

Figure 7 Pregnancy-associated progesterone production by cultured cumulus cells (progesterone/cumulus–oocyte complex/24 h). Control: 7.5 nmol/l

throughout. Some evidence suggests that progesterone production *in vitro* peaks at the equivalent of 6–8 weeks' gestation and subsequently falls (Figure 7); however, in other cycles progesterone concentrations continued to rise throughout the first-trimester period (author's unpublished observation).

Cumulus and corona cells were also shown to produce oestradiol in culture. The role of oestrogens in human implantation has not been established. It has been shown in rodents that relatively low concentrations of oestrogens acting upon a progesterone-primed endometrium create a 24-hour implantation window[16]. The observation that human cumulus and corona cells produce oestradiol *in vitro* leads to the suggestion that these cells are a source of oestradiol which may be involved in the creation of a similar implantation window.

Plasma oestradiol concentrations in the follicular phase for the Coat-a-Count assay lie in the range 0.6–1.0 nmol/l per oocyte. Thus, both corona and cumulus oestradiol production levels, in the range 0.3–3.2 nmol/l per COC/24 h, are capable of producing a localized, physiologically significant effect. Preliminary observations on oestradiol concentrations in pregnancy-related cultures suggest increasing concentrations from day 1 of culture, reaching a peak after 5–6 days' culture. Thereafter, oestradiol concentrations begin to fall, in some cases to their

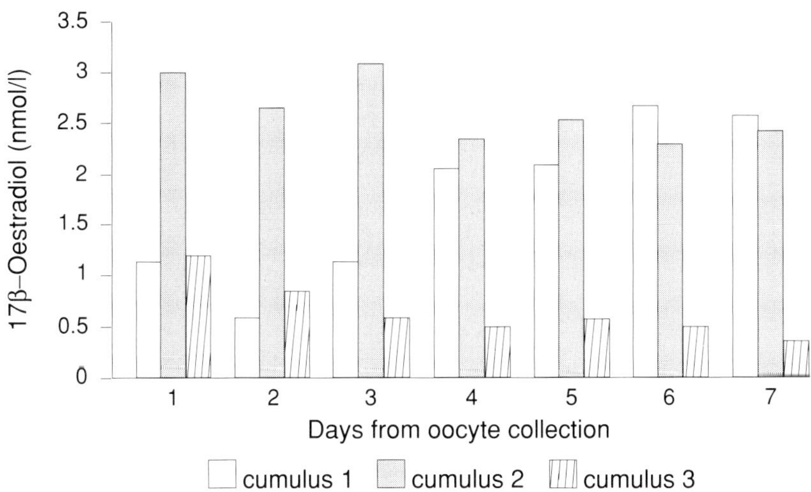

Figure 8 17β-Oestradiol production by cultured cumulus cells: 17β-oestradiol per cumulus–oocyte complex per 24 h. Cumulus 1, pregnancy-related; cumulus 2 + 3, associated with failed *in vitro* fertilization. Control assays: cumulus 1, 0.6 nmol/l; cumulus 2+3, 0.22–0.4 nmol/l

original level (Figure 8). Oestradiol concentrations in non-pregnant cycles were of the same magnitude or greater but did not display the same time-course distribution (Figure 8). Cultured cumulus and corona cells continue to produce oestradiol *in vitro* for up to 80 days when cultures were discarded.

Immunosuppression

The production of a soluble, embryo-derived immunosuppressant has been demonstrated by the capacity of culture supernatant to suppress lymphocyte transformation in the presence of a mitogenic agent such as phytohaemagglutinin or concanavalin A[17]. We have evidence that supernatant from cumulus and corona culture, sampled on consecutive days for up to 6 days after embryo transfer, has the capacity to suppress lymphocyte transformation in the presence of phytohaemagglutinin (author and colleagues' unpublished observations).

Table 2 The suppression of lymphocyte transformation in venous blood culture in the presence of phytohaemagglutinin (PHA) by supernatant from cumulus and corona cultures. Lymphocyte transformation measured as 'large unclassified cells' (LUC) as a percentage of the white cell population

	LUC (%)
Control cultures	
no PHA	< 0.6
plus PHA	18–30
Test cultures (+PHA)	
plus cumulus supernatant	6–11
plus corona supernatant	4.5–7.5

Evidence for lymphocyte transformation following incubation with PHA (Murex Diagnostics Ltd., Dartford, UK) was demonstrated by the presence of 18–30% 'large unclassified cells' (LUC) in a full blood count assay on a Technicon Haematology System. Where lymphocytes were not exposed to phytohaemagglutinin, then LUC comprised < 0.6% of the white cell population. The addition of supernatant from cumulus and corona culture systems to lymphocytes cultured with phytohaemagglutinin resulted in a 66% and 75% suppression of transformation, respectively (Table 2).

Immunocytochemistry has shown that cumulus and corona cells *in vitro* express the complement inhibiting proteins decay accelerating factor and complement regulatory protein CD59 within 24 h of oocyte collection and after approximately 14 days of culture (author and colleagues' unpublished data).

DISCUSSION

It is becoming increasingly evident that cumulus tissue expresses a number of functions with the potential to influence the processes which govern oocyte maturation, ovulation, fertilization and implantation. Intrafollicular materials are transported to the oocyte via the cumulus mass[18], secretions of the cumulus have been shown to alter sperm motility[19] and the activity of granulosa–lutein cells in mice has been shown to be modulated by the oocyte; oocytectomy resulting in a 17–36% increase in progesterone production by cumulus in the presence of follicle stimulating hormone (FSH)[20]. Thus, cumulus progesterone production *in vivo* may be downregulated by the oocyte until the cells are dispersed by the action of spermatozoa.

It is appropriate here to distinguish between granulosa–lutein cells and cells of the cumulus/corona. Fish and colleagues[12] showed that granulosa–lutein cells produce progesterone *in vitro* for up to 4 days from oocyte collection and for up to 14 days when cultured in the presence of LH or FSH. After 14 days they were unable to stimulate the cells further. Our evidence demonstrates that cumulus/corona cells have the capacity to maintain progesterone production *in vitro* for up to 80 days in the absence of exogenous stimulation. This difference in the steroidogenic capacity of the cells is illustrative of the differences in the cell lines.

Events *in vivo* following ovulation result in the cumulus being dispersed in the ampullary region of the Fallopian tube by the action of sper- matozoa. The corona, however, would be retained by the embryo. To extrapolate from the murine model[20] the removal of the influence of the oocyte would allow progesterone production to achieve its full potential. In IVF–ET, however, both events are disrupted. The cumulus is dispersed *in vitro* and becomes lost to the system, and the corona is disrupted to allow the oocyte to be assessed for evidence of fertilization.

The adhesive property of cumulus cells, which has been demonstrated *in vitro*, would (following their dispersal by spermatozoa) allow adhesion to the tube lining and subsequent proliferation and steroid production. In this context the distribution of progesterone receptors in the female system is significant. The highest concentrations of progesterone receptors are found in the ampullary region of the Fallopian tube and the fundus of the uterus[21]. These receptors are, therefore, concentrated at or close to the site of progesterone production by cumulus and corona cells which we have shown are capable of producing local concentrations far in excess of that in plasma at the same time. It may also be significant that most embryos implant in the fundus where high concentrations of progesterone receptors have been identified.

It has been demonstrated that the application of exogenous proges- terone in advance of ovulation results in significantly increased pregnancy rates[22] from IVF. Additionally, the intravaginal administration of micronized progesterone has resulted in a significant reduction in abortion rates[23] from IVF. Thus, cumulus progesterone production in close proximity to the uterus may be more significant to endometrial priming than plasma progesterone. Additionally, the administration of exogenous progesterone in IVF at this time may clearly compensate for the loss of progesterone production by the cumulus.

Because of the difficulty of obtaining material from the implantation period in primates, it has not been established whether oestrogen is necessary to the implantation process. However, it has been suggested that primate blastocysts or endometrium may synthesize oestrogens which could act locally to facilitate implantation[24]. The production of oestradiol by cumulus and corona could serve this and a number of other functions. It would facilitate the priming of oestrogen receptors in the ampulla and fundus and the interaction between oestrogen and progesterone may be responsible for the transfer of the embryo into the uterus – progesterone acting to retain the embryo at the ampullary–isthmic junction, while a sufficient pulse of oestradiol may be required to expel the embryo into the uterus. Thus, an abnormality of the oestrogen:progesterone ratio in the tubal environment at this time may interfere with timed transfer of embryo into the uterus or asynchrony of endometrial maturation.

Oestradiol production by these cells may have further significance for implantation since they have the potential to provide a pulse of oestradiol which may be necessary to create an implantation window.

It has further been suggested that oestradiol contributes to implantation by facilitating embryo hatching through zona thinning[25]. The corona cells, because of their intimate contact with the zona and their potential to produce oestradiol, may clearly contribute to the hatching process. The disruption of the corona in IVF may explain the phenomenon of zona tanning which develops with time in culture and may also explain the success of implantation following assisted hatching[26], where the puncture of the zona may compensate for the removal of corona cells.

The evidence for the steroidogenic properties of these cells suggests that some of the failure of implantation recorded in IVF may be a direct consequence of technique, i.e. the discarding of cumulus cells following insemination and the disruption of the corona. These actions could result in a steroid deficiency/imbalance at this critical time for endometrial receptivity, and an alteration in the embryonic micro-environment.

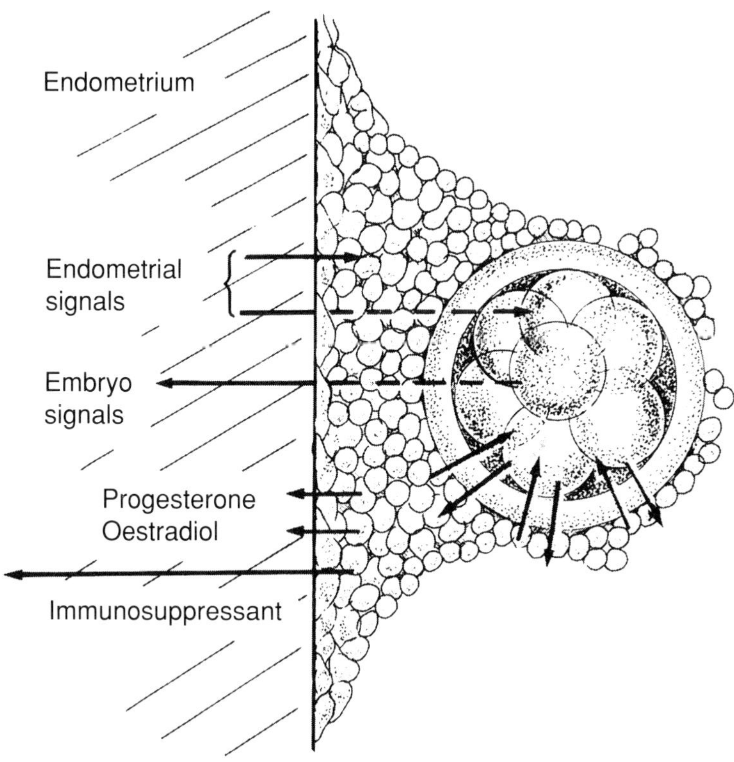

Figure 9 Diagrammatic representation of the potential contribution of corona cells at the foeto-maternal interface in the peri-implantation period

The observation that cumulus and corona cells have the capacity to produce a soluble immunosuppressant *in vitro* is further supportive of the hypothesis that they have the potential to influence implantation. Whereas the production of a soluble immunosuppressant by cumulus cells could exert a generalized effect on the endometrium, the potential contribution of the corona is more significant. These cells remain in intimate contact with the embryo and have the capacity to attach the embryo *in vitro* to the culture surface and undergo subsequent proliferation. Thus, it has been suggested[14,15] that these cells could, *in vivo*, attach the embryo at the implantation site (Figure 9).

The presence of a corona cell layer at the foeto-maternal interface could promote a number of functions. Being maternal in origin the cells would not stimulate an antigenic response in the endometrium at the time of attachment. This would not explain the success of embryo donation. The cells, however, may play a significant role in immunosuppression in the peri-implantation period. Having assumed an intimate attachment with the endometrium they could form a buffer, serving to mask the embryonic genome from the maternal system whilst exposing the endometrium to a soluble immunosuppressant. This could act on the endometrium at the implantation site in advance of invasion by the embryo and prepare the implantation site. These cells could also serve to transmit signals from foetus to endometrium and vice versa while continuing to express their own signals. Indirect evidence in support of this theory is provided by the observation that exogenous immunosuppressants increase pregnancy rates in IVF-related treatments where there is a major disruption of these cells. It has been suggested that those IVF-related techniques which entail puncture of the zona compromise the immunosuppressive capacity of the embryo and that exogenous immunosuppressants which compensate for this event lead to increased pregnancy rates[27]. Since these techniques invariably involve a major disruption to the corona layer, it may be postulated that the compromised immunosuppression reflects the removal of these cells, rather than zona puncture.

The observation that cumulus and corona cells maintain their steroidogenic capacity *in vitro* through the equivalent of the first trimester of pregnancy leads to the suggestion that they may persist at the foeto-maternal interface, possibly exerting a paracrine effect on the trophoblast in respect of steroidogenesis. Further, indirect evidence for the potential of these cells to influence the implantation process is provided by a comparison of implantation rates from gamete intrafallopian transfer (GIFT) and IVF. Thus, Mills and colleagues[28] showed, in a prospective randomized study, that whereas pregnancy rates from GIFT and IVF did not differ significantly, the implantation rates from GIFT treatments were significantly greater than IVF. Since these results were generated by the same centre, one must assume that the only contributing differences were techniques relating to *in vitro* culture. The reduced implantation rates from IVF may, therefore, have been a reflection of the depletion of cumulus and corona.

These observations offer ovarian cell function as an alternative, non-invasive means of evaluating embryo quality and identify the need for further research to clarify the role of these cells in human reproduction.

ACKNOWLEDGEMENTS

I wish to acknowledge the considerable contribution of Dr Catherine Wells, Unit for Assisted Reproduction, University Hospital of Wales, Cardiff, in respect of cell culture techniques and assistance with this manuscript. I also wish to acknowledge Mrs D.E. Davies, Department of Obstetrics and Gynaecology; Dr I. Rooney, Dept of Biochemistry; Mr Kevin Williams, Department of Haematology; and the Department of Medical Illustration, University of Wales College of Medicine, Cardiff for their assistance with steroid assays, immunocytochemistry, haematology and photographic work, respectively. I also wish to thank Mrs S.M. Walker, Director of Assisted Reproduction for her support of this ongoing research project.

REFERENCES

1. O'Neill, C. (1985). Thrombocytopoenia is an initial maternal response to fertilisation in mice. *J. Reprod. Fertil.*, **73**, 567–77
2. Lenton, E.A., Neal, L.M. and Sulaiman, R. (1982). Plasma concentrations of human chorionic gonadotrophin from the time of implantation until the second week of pregnancy. *Fertil. Steril.*, **37**, 773–8
3. Shulman, A., Ben-Nun, I., Ghetler, Y., Kaneti, H., Shilon, M. and Beyth, Y. (1993). Relationship between embryo morphology and implantation rate after *in vitro* fertilisation treatment in conception cycles. *Fertil. Steril.*, **60**, 123–6
4. Plachot, M. (1992). Viability of preimplantation embryos. *Baillières Clin. Obstet. Gynaecol.*, **6**, 327–38
5. Leese, H.J. and Barton, A.M. (1984). Pyruvate and glucose uptake by mouse ova and preimplantation embryos. *J. Reprod. Fertil.*, **72**, 9–13
6. Leese, H.J., Hooper, M.A.K., Edwards, R.G. and Ashwood-Smith, M.J. (1986). Uptake of pyruvate by early human embryos determined by a non-invasive technique. *Hum. Reprod.*, **1**, 181–2
7. Human Fertilisation and Embryology Authority (1993). *Annual Report*, London: HMSO
8. Alberman, E., Creasy, M., Elliot, M. and Spicer, C. (1976). Maternal factors associated with foetal chromosome anomalies in spontaneous abortions. *Br. J. Obstet. Gynaecol.*, **83**, 621–7
9. Carr, D.H. (1967). Chromosome anomalies as a cause of spontaneous abortion. *Am. J. Obstet. Gynecol.*, **97**, 283–93

10. Michael, A.E., Gregory, L., Walker, S.M., Antoniw, J.W., Shaw, R.W., Edwards, C.R.W. and Cooke, B.A. (1993). Ovarian 11β-hydroxysteroid dehydrogenase: potential predictor of conception by *in vitro* fertilisation and embryo transfer. *Lancet*, **342**, 711–12

11. Gregory, L., Booth, A.D., Wells, C.W. and Walker, S.M. (1994). A study of the cumulus–corona complex in *in-vitro* fertilisation and embryo transfer: a prognostic indicator of the failure of implantation. *Hum. Reprod.*, **9**, 1308–17

12. Fish, B., Margara, R.A., Winston, R.M.L. and Hillier, S.G. (1989). Cellular basis of luteal steroidogenesis in the human ovary. *J. Endocrinol.*, **122**, 303–11

13. Csapo, A.I., Pulkinnen, M.O., Rutter, B., Sauvage, J.P. and Wiest, W.G. (1972). The significance of the human corpus luteum in pregnancy maintenance. *Am. J. Obstet. Gynecol.*, **112**, 1061–7

14. Gregory, L., Wells, C., Davies, D.E., Vine, S.J. and Walker, S.M. (1994). The role of ovarian cells in the peri-implantation processes in human IVF–ET. *Br. J. Obstet. Gynaecol.*, **101**, 732–3

15. Gregory, L., Wells, C., Vine, S.J., Davies, D.E. and Walker, S.M. (1994). The role of human ovarian cells in the peri-implantation process and early pregnancy. *Contemp. Rev. Obstet. Gynaecol.*, **6**, 195–200

16. Findlay, J.K. (1983). The endocrinology of the preimplantation period. In Martini, L. and James, V. (eds.) *Pregnancy and Parturition, Current Topics in Endocrinology*. Vol.4, pp. 35–67. (New York: Academic Press)

17. Jones, K.P., Warnock, S.H., Urry, R.L., Edwin, S.S. and Mitchell, M.D. (1992). Immunosuppressive activity and alpha interferon concentrations in human embryo culture media as an index of potential for successful implantation. *Fertil. Steril.*, **57**, 637–40

18. Moor, R.M., Smith, M.W. and Dawson, R.M. (1980). Measurement of intracellular coupling between oocytes and cumulus cells using intracellular markers. *Exp. Cell Res.*, **126**, 15–29

19. Tesarik, J., Mendoza Oltras, C. and Testart, J. Effect of human cumulus oophorus on movement characteristics of human capacitated spermatozoa. *J. Reprod. Fertil.*, **88**, 665–75

20. Vanderhyden, B.C. and Armstrong, D.T. (1989). Role of cumulus cells and serum in the *in vitro* maturation, fertilisation and subsequent development of rat oocytes. *Biol. Reprod.*, **40**, 720–8

21. Coppens, M.T., de Boever, J.G., Dhont, M.A., Serreyn, R.F., Vandekerckhove, D.A. and Roels, H.J. (1993). Topographical distribution of oestrogen and progesterone receptors in the human endometrium and Fallopian tube. An immunocytochemical study. *Histochemistry*, **99**, 127–31

22. Ben-Nun, I., Ghetler, Y., Jaffe, R., Siegal, A., Kaneti, H. and Fejgin, M. (1992). Effect of preovulatory progesterone administration on the endome-

trial maturation and implantation rate after *in vitro* fertilisation and embryo transfer. *Fertil. Steril.*, **53**, 276–81

23. Smitz, J., Devroey, P., Fauger, B., Bourgain, C., Camus, M. and Van Steirteghem, A.C. (1992). A prospective randomised comparison of intramuscular or intravaginal natural progesterone as a luteal phase and early pregnancy supplement. *Hum. Reprod.*, **7**, 168–75

24. Findlay, J.K. (1984). Implantation and early pregnancy. In Trounson, A. and Wood, C. (eds.) *In Vitro Fertilization and Embryo Transfer*, pp. 57–72, (Edinburgh: Churchill Livingstone)

25. Klopper, A. (1985). Steroids in pregnancy. In Shearman, R.P. (ed.) *Clinical Reproductive Endocrinology*, pp.209–23 (Edinburgh: Churchill Livingstone)

26. Alikani, M. and Cohen, J. (1992). Advances in micromanipulation of gametes and embryos. Assisted fertilisation and hatching. *Arch. Pathol. Lab. Med.*, **116**, 373–8

27. Cohen, J., Malter, H., Elsner, C., Kort, H., Massey, J. and Mayer, M.P. (1990). Immunosuppression supports implantation of zona pellucida dissected human embryos. *Fertil. Steril.*, **53**, 625–55

28. Mills, M.S., Eddowes, H.A., Cahill, D.J., Fahy, U.M., Abuzeid, M.I., McDermott, A. and Hull, M. (1992). A prospective controlled randomised study of *in vitro* fertilisation, gamete intrafallopian transfer and intrauterine insemination combined with superovulation. *Hum. Reprod.*, **7**, 490–4

29. Michael, A.E., Gregory, L., Piercy, E.C., Antonin, J.W., Shaw, R.W., Edwards, C.R.W. and Cooke, B.A. (1993). Clinical correlates of ovarian 11 beta-hydroxysteroid dehydrogenase (11βHSD) activity in patients undergoing *in vitro* fertilisation–embryo transfer (IVF–ET). *J. Endocrinol.*, **139** (suppl.) abstr. 028

4

Clinical monitoring for *in vitro* fertilization

R.G. Forman and S.A. Adeaga

INTRODUCTION

Clinical monitoring for *in vitro* fertilization (IVF) is an area where the art and the science of ovulation stimulation are closely interwoven. This is due in part to the natural reluctance of many IVF centres to experiment with or change a successful formula. Others would argue that this is an area that has not been subject to the harsh glare of scientific investigation.

There has been considerable evolution in ovulation stimulation proto-cols for IVF over the past 15 years. The early natural cycles were followed by clomiphene stimulation, then gonadotrophin stimulation and now the association of gonadotrophin releasing hormone agonists (GnRHa) and gonadotrophins. However, there has been a slower evolution in moni-toring techniques and some of the basic principles of monitoring which were first elucidated in natural cycles have been applied uncritically to modern methods of stimulation. The pharmacophysiology of gonadotro-phin stimulation following pituitary down-regulation with GnRHa is far removed from our understanding of pituitary–ovarian relationships in the natural cycle. For example, there is a near perfect correlation between the mean follicular diameter of the dominant follicle and serum oestradiol in natural cycles[1]. In stimulated cycles this simple relationship is lost[2,3], presumably because the largest follicle is not necessarily the most oestrogenic. Ovulation has been reported to occur at a mean follicular diameter of 20–27 mm in natural cycles, 15–24 mm in clomiphene-stimulated and 13–30 mm in gonadotrophin-stimulated cycles[4].

45

AIMS OF CLINICAL MONITORING FOR IVF

In 1986 Kerin and Warnes defined the aim of monitoring in IVF cycles to 'determine the magnitude and normality of the endocrine and growth response of the selected cohort of follicles which have been recruited during the early follicular phase and to determine the start of a luteinizing hormone (LH) surge or the optimal time for human chorionic gonadotrophin (hCG) administration'[5]. This definition is now largely outdated, as the vast majority of IVF cycles are performed using protocols incorporating GnRHa, and a spontaneous LH surge is no longer a threat to the IVF cycle. It has, however, been replaced by the spectre of ovarian hyperstimulation syndrome (OHSS). The aims of clinical monitoring today can be best summarized as follows:

(1) To determine the optimum time for hCG administration.

(2) To predict and, therefore, prevent the development of severe ovarian hyperstimulation syndrome.

(3) To identify poor responder cycles with a view to improving the response or cancelling the cycle.

MODALITIES OF CYCLE MONITORING FOR IVF

Both hormonal and ultrasonographic criteria have been used to monitor the IVF cycle.

Endocrine assessment

17β-oestradiol

Serum 17β-oestradiol measurements are routine although the frequency with which they are used varies greatly between centres. Some units never measure 17β-oestradiol but rely solely on ultrasound measurement of follicular diameter. Others measure oestradiol levels on a daily basis. Jones and colleagues[6] were the first group to propose that serial oestradiol measurements correlate with IVF outcome, by relating the oestradiol pattern in the terminal phases of follicular growth to the pregnancy rate. Others confirmed these findings subsequently, but this work was all performed in cycles stimulated by gonadotrophins with or without

Table 1 Influence of the oestradiol pattern on IVF results; hCG, human chorionic gonadotrophin

	Oestradiol pattern			
	A	*G*	*D*	*E*
Number of cycles	175	58	27	13
Oestradiol (pg/ml) at time of hCG★	933 ± 609	1249 ± 992	467 ± 352	1035 ± 1548
Oocytes per cycle★	6.73 ± 3.78	7.15 ± 4.68	4.12 ± 2.85	6.00 ± 7.29
Embryos per cycle★	4.64 ± 3.53	4.94 ± 4.26	3.00 ± 2.66	5.09 ± 6.50
Pregnancy rate (%)	35	38	33	39

★ values are means ± SD

clomiphene citrate[7,8]. Recently, we repeated this work in patients having first IVF cycles stimulated with human menopausal gonadotrophin (hMG) following preliminary down-regulation with buserelin[9]. The results are shown in Table 1. Patterns A and G (in which oestradiol increased daily until the time of hCG) were the most favourable patterns in the previous studies, whereas patterns D and E (in which a fall in oestradiol was recorded at some time prior to hCG) were the least favourable (in fact, Jones and colleagues[6] observed no pregnancies with the latter two patterns). As can be seen in Table 1, using ovulation stimulation protocols as currently performed, the pattern of oestradiol in the terminal phase of follicular growth bore no relationship to the IVF outcome and pregnancy rates. In the same study the oestradiol levels achieved on the day that hCG was administered to trigger ovulation were compared to the outcome of IVF. Table 2 shows that higher oestradiol levels were associated with the recovery of more oocytes from more follicles; hence a greater number of embryos were obtained in the presence of high oestradiol levels. Significantly, however, the pregnancy rate per cycle did not correlate at all with the oestradiol level, because even in patients with oestradiol levels < 500 pg/ml on the day of hCG administration, three embryos were obtained. On the basis of these results, the efficacy of oestradiol monitoring to determine the optimum time for hCG administration must be strongly questioned.

Table 2 Influence of the height of the oestradiol (E_2) response on IVF outcome; hCG, human chorionic gonadotrophin

	E_2 on day of hCG (pg/ml)				
	≤ 500	501–1000	1001–1500	1501–2000	≥ 2000
Number of cycles	66	120	59	41	29
Oocytes per cycle*	3.66 ± 2.39	5.87 ± 2.53	8.41 ± 4.40	10.92 ± 4.20	12.82 ± 5.48
Embryos per cycle*	2.72 ± 2.28	4.31 ± 2.60	5.78 ± 4.00	5.40 ± 5.17	8.11 ± 6.20
Pregnancy rate (%)	33	38	36	27	31

*values are means ± SD

An interesting study was reported recently by Tan and co-workers[10], in which they decided on the optimal timing for hCG administration based on their conventional criteria. These were: the presence of a leading follicle of 18 mm and two other follicles greater than 14 mm, with an appropriate level of oestradiol. They randomly allocated some of their patients to receive hCG at this time. Others were given their hCG 24 or 48 h later. As might be expected, there were significant differences in the oestradiol levels at the time the hCG was administered but no difference in any of the IVF results, including the pregnancy rate[10].

Luteinizing hormone

In the past, other hormone measurements have been made in monitoring IVF cycles. In particular, prior to the adoption of GnRHa down-regulation protocols, LH levels were ascertained both to exclude high baseline LH levels, which are known to be detrimental to IVF outcome[11,12], and also to identify the onset of an LH surge. In natural cycles LH was measured in urine, 2–4 hourly[13]. Testart and colleagues[14] developed the concept of the LH surge-initiating rise in which a serum LH value exceeding 180%

of the mean of the previous four values was counted as the beginning of a surge. This all became redundant with the adoption of down-regulation protocols.

Other endocrine parameters

Progesterone has been used as an indicator of premature LH surges[15], but again this is not relevant to the use of modern stimulation protocols. Finally, inhibin has been investigated as a method of assessing ovarian function in women undergoing hMG stimulation for IVF following GnRHa down-regulation[16]. In one study, inhibin levels correlated well with oestradiol levels during stimulation and on the day of hCG administration. Inhibin levels were also seen to correlate with the number of preovulatory follicles on ultrasound. However, inhibin offers no advantages over oestradiol measurements in ovulation monitoring.

Ultrasound assessment

Follicular diameter

Ultrasound monitoring of ovulation stimulation generally involves measuring the number of ovarian follicles and their mean diameter. Some IVF programmes perform follicular ultrasound as the sole method of monitoring, although more frequently both follicular ultrasound and serum oestradiol measurements are performed. Various formulae have been used to calculate the appropriate time to administer hCG − for example, the oestradiol value per follicle having attained a defined size[17]. Alternatively, a threshold oestradiol level, obtained in the presence of a certain number of follicles of a defined size, may be specified[18]. As mentioned above, however, the assumed relationship between follicle size and oestradiol level is less accurate using GnRHa. Consider the frequently observed situation in patients with polycystic ovaries, in which very high oestradiol levels are achieved associated with the presence of many very small follicles.

Ultrasound monitoring of ovarian follicles is now mostly carried out using the vaginal route. In a comparison between transabdominal and transvaginal follicular scanning Belaisch-Allart and co-workers[19] reported that both the number of follicles seen was higher and the recorded follicular diameter was greater using the vaginal route. These authors

Table 3 Influence of the number of preovulatory follicles on day 0 on IVF outcome; hCG, human chorionic gonadotrophin

	Number of follicles > 14 mm diameter on day 0				
	≤ 2	3–4	5–6	7–8	≥ 9
Number of cycles	25	19	102	59	35
Oestradiol (pg/ml) at time of hCG*	401 ± 224	662 ± 384	1025 ± 476	1495 ± 711	1713 ± 988
Oocytes per cycle*	3.41 ± 3.19	4.61 ± 2.35	7.26 ± 3.20	10.14 ± 5.63	11.63 ± 4.43
Embryos per cycle*	2.50 ± 3.08	3.68 ± 2.22	4.99 ± 3.30	6.64 ± 5.40	7.81 ± 5.47
Pregnancy rate (%)	52	33	37	34	20

*values are means ± SD

drew attention to the fact that the criteria for hCG injection needed to be adjusted when teams changed from abdominal to vaginal scanning.

In our study described above we were interested in assessing the reliability of follicular scanning as a method of predicting IVF outcome[9]. Table 3 shows the relationship between the number of follicles of 15 mm or greater on the day of ovulation induction with hCG compared to IVF outcome. It was very surprising to discover that the group with the highest pregnancy rate (greater than 50% per cycle commenced) were those with only one or two preovulatory follicles. However, a mean of 3.4 oocytes was obtained even in this group. Mature oocytes are therefore harvestable from follicles < 15 mm in diameter. The pregnancy rate was lowest in those patients with many follicles. The diameter of the leading follicle was unrelated to outcome (Table 4). This led to the conclusion that follicular scanning was a poor predictor of IVF success, and also raised the question of the accuracy of follicular ultrasound measurements. The results of an endocrine measurement can be stated with a high

Table 4 Influence of the diameter of the leading follicle on day 0 on IVF outcome; hCG, human chorionic gonadotrophin

	Mean diameter of largest follicle on day of hCG				
	15–16 mm	*17–18 mm*	*19–20 mm*	*21–22 mm*	*> 23 mm*
Number of cycles	27	135	91	32	25
Oestradiol (pg/ml) at time of hCG[A]	988 ± 556	1005 ± 654	1069 ± 815	1001 ± 626	1183 ± 728
Oocytes per cycle*	7.88 ± 4.06	7.10 ± 4.65	7.08 ± 4.24	7.23 ± 3.91	7.70 ± 6.29
Embryos per cycle*	5.77 ± 3.55	5.02 ± 4.11	4.68 ± 4.04	5.27 ± 4.02	5.35 ± 4.97
Pregnancy rate (%)	33	33	39	31	28

*values are means ± SD

degree of accuracy, and variation around the mean can be calculated. The same cannot be said for ultrasound assessment of follicular size, as there is no 'gold standard' for comparison – the 'true' follicular diameter is unknown. This is of practical relevance because important clinical management decisions are taken based on these results. We undertook a study to quantify accuracy and reproducibility of transvaginal follicular scanning in IVF[20]. This study involved four skilled observers, each making two independent measurements of the same follicle in a stimulated IVF cycle. A total of 20 follicles was studied. Following statistical analysis of the results it was possible to calculate both within-observer and between-observer variation. For a follicle of 15 mm diameter, the 95% confidence interval for a single observer is 13–17 mm; between observers, the interval is 12–18 mm. It was relevant that larger follicles were associated with the greatest measurement error; this is a significant range and could partly explain the poor predictive value of follicular size and IVF outcome.

Endometrial thickness

Another ultrasound parameter suggested for cycle monitoring is measurement of endometrial thickness and reflectivity. Thickness of the endometrium correlates with circulating oestradiol levels, but there are conflicting views in the literature about how this relates to IVF outcome. Some authors have described no difference in endometrial thickness in those achieving pregnancy compared to non-conceptual IVF cycles[21,22]. Others have noted a significant correlation between thickness and occurrence of pregnancy[23].

Endometrial reflectivity

The pattern of endometrial reflectivity at ultrasound examination has also been described. Two basic patterns have been noted: Type A, consisting of a homogeneous hyperechogenic appearance, and Type B, which has a mixed appearance, with an outer hyperechogenic layer and an inner hypoechogenic layer. A third pattern, Type C, describes the presence of a fluid-filled ring in the endometrial cavity. Different nomenclatures have been used. For example, patterns A and B have also been described as patterns I and II[24]. There is similar disagreement on the predictive ability of endometrial pattern to predict cycle outcome. Sher and colleagues[24] reported optimal pregnancy rates in thick pattern II endometrium, but poor results in thin pattern II and all pattern I endometrium. Ueno and co-workers[25] reported no pregnancies with pattern A endometrium. Khalifa and associates[26], on the other hand, found no correlation between endometrial pattern and outcome of the IVF cycle.

The qualitative interpretation of endometrial ultrasound is a subjective assessment and it is perhaps not surprising that there is disagreement in the literature upon the importance of this sign in predicting IVF outcome. Currently, this particular measurement only has a small role in monitoring the IVF cycle. The use of Doppler ultrasonography to assess ovarian response to stimulation is discussed in Chapter 6.

PREDICTION OF OHSS

Ovarian hyperstimulation syndrome is probably the most serious complication of *in vitro* fertilization, both in terms of the severity of the disorder and its relatively high incidence. The condition is reviewed in Chapter 8, but there is total agreement that prevention is better than cure. It is of the utmost importance that IVF practitioners have protocols to identify patients who are at high risk of developing the severe form of OHSS. The cycle can then be cancelled or managed differently from the normal situation.

Unfortunately there is no universal agreement on the parameters of follicular response that are predictive for OHSS. In our own analysis of eight cases of severe OHSS, all patients had oestradiol levels in excess of 2000 pg/ml in the presence of 15 or more follicles ≥ 12 mm. The sensitivity (proportion of true positives correctly identified) of these parameters as a screening procedure was 100% and its specificity (proportion of true negatives correctly identified), 88%. However, only 1 in 4 patients who fulfil these criteria would develop severe OHSS[27]. Golan and colleagues[28] confirmed the importance of oestradiol levels > 2000 pg/ml at the time of hCG administration in patients developing the severe form of OHSS. Patients who are known to have polycystic ovaries[29]. or who have the typical 'necklace sign' on transvaginal scanning of their ovaries, are at particular risk of OHSS[30]. Blankstein and co-workers[31] indicated that the number of small follicles (< 9 mm diameter) on the day of hCG administration also correlated with an increased risk of OHSS.

LOW RESPONDERS

One aspect of monitoring of IVF cycles which is certainly important is the ability to identify those patients who fail to respond to ovulation stimulation. The cycles of women who show no follicular activity after hMG stimulation need to be either cancelled or modified by increasing the dose of stimulation. There are no data to show whether cycle cancellation, or trying to rescue the cycle by increasing the dose of hMG, is the best strategy. Knowledge of early follicular phase follicle stimulating hormone (FSH) levels is important, as patients with raised FSH can be predicted to be poor responders, and a high dose of hMG can be prescribed for the treatment cycle. More controversial is the management strategy when there is some follicular response but this response is considered to be suboptimal. Our own view is based on the work discussed above showing that pregnancy rates correlate poorly with both oestradiol levels and follicle numbers. Therefore, even if only a small number of preovulatory follicles is present, it may be preferable to induce ovulation with hCG rather than cancel the cycle[9].

CONCLUSION

Some form of clinical monitoring of IVF cycles is invariably performed. The rationale behind monitoring is debatable; it has an important role in helping to identify patients who may be at risk of developing severe OHSS and, at the other end of the spectrum, in identifying those patients who have completely failed to respond to stimulation. Between these two extremes there is little evidence that current methods of cycle monitoring are effective at predicting the outcome of the IVF cycle. This observation would suggest that a minimal level of monitoring only is appropriate. Units performing intensive cycle monitoring need to justify this approach on the basis of improved pregnancy rates, compared to the minimalist approach.

REFERENCES

1. Hackeloer, B.J., Fleming, R., Robinson, H.P., Adam, A.H and Coutts, J.R.T. (1979). Correlation of ultrasonographic and endocrinologic assessment of human follicular development. *Am. J. Obstet. Gynecol.*, **135**, 122–8
2. Sallan, H.N., Marinho, A.O., Collins, W.P., Rodeck, C.H. and Cambell, S. (1982). Monitoring gonadotrophin therapy by real time ultrasonic scanning of ovarian follicles. *Br. J. Obstet. Gynaecol.*, **89**, 155–9
3. Mantzavinos, T., Garcia, J.E. and Jones, H.W. (1983). Ultrasound measurement of ovarian follicles stimulated by human gonadotrophins for oocyte recovery and *in vitro* fertilisation. *Fertil. Steril.*, **40**, 461–5
4. Tarlatzis, B.C., Laufer, N. and DeCherney, A.H. (1984). The use of ovarian ultrasonography in monitoring ovulation induction. *J. In Vitro Fertil. Embryo Transfer*, **1**, 226–32
5. Kerin, J.F. and Warnes, G.M. (1986). Monitoring of ovarian response to stimulation on *in vitro* fertilization cycles. *Clin. Obstet. Gynaecol.*, **29**, 158–70
6. Jones, H.W. J., Acosta, A., Andrews, M.C., Garcia, J.E., Jones, G.S., Mantzavinos, T., McDowell, J., Sandow, B., Veeeck, L., Whibley, T.,

Wilkes, C. and Wright, G. (1983). The importance of the follicular phase and success or failure in *in vitro* fertilization. *Fertil. Steril.*, **40**, 317–21

7. Dor, J., Rudak, E., Maschiach, S., Nebel, L., Serr, D.M. and Goldman, B. (1986). Periovulatory 17-beta estradiol changes and embryo morphological features in conception and non-conceptional cycles after human *in vitro* fertilization. *Fertil. Steril.*, **45**, 63–8

8. Laufer, N., DeCherney, A.H., Tarlatzis, B.C. and Naftolin, F. (1986). The association between preovulatory 17-beta estradiol pattern and conception in human menopausal gonadotrophin, human chorionic gonadotrophin stimulation. *Fertil. Steril.*, **46**, 73–6

9. Forman, R., Robinson, J., Egan, D., Ross, C., Gosden, B. and Barlow, D. (1991). Follicular monitoring and outcome of *in vitro* fertilization in gonadotrophin releasing hormone agonists treated cycles. *Fertil. Steril.*, **55**, 567–73

10. Tan, S.L., Balen, A., El Hussein, E., Mills, C., Campbell, S., Yovich, J. and Jacobs, H.S. (1992). A prospective randomised study of the optimum timing of human chorionic gonadotrophin administration after pituitary desensitization in *in vitro* fertilization. *Fertil. Steril.*, **57**, 1259–64

11. Stanger, J.D. and Yovich, J.L. (1985). Reduced *in vitro* fertilization of human oocytes from patients with raised basal luteinizing hormone levels during the follicular phase. *Br. J. Obstet. Gynaecol.*, **92**, 385–93

12. Howles, C.M., Macnamee, M.C. and Edwards, R.G. (1987). Follicular development and early luteal function of conception and non-conception cycles after human *in vitro* fertilization: endocrine correlates. *Hum. Reprod.*, **2**, 17–21

13. Edwards, R.G., Steptoe, P.C. and Purdy, J.M. (1980). Establishing full term human pregnancies using cleaving embryos grown *in vitro*. *Br. J. Obstet. Gynaecol.*, **87**, 737–56

14. Testart, J., Frydman, R., Feinstein, M.C., Thebault, A., Roger, M. and Scholler, R. (1981). Interpretation of plasma luteinizing hormone assay for the collection of mature oocytes from women: definition of a luteinizing hormone surge-initiating rise. *Fertil. Steril.* **36**, 50–4

15. Feldberg, D., Goldman, G.A., Ashkenazi, J., Dicker, D., Shelef, M. and Goldman, J.A. (1989). The impact of high progesterone levels in the follicular phase of *in vitro* fertilization (IVF) cycles: a comparative study. *J. In Vitro Fertil. Embryo Transfer*, **6**, 11–14

16. Matson, P.L., Morris, I.D., Sun, J.G., Ibrahim, Z.H. and Lieberman, B.A. (1991). Serum inhibin as an index of ovarian function in women undergoing pituitary suppression and ovarian stimulation in an *in vitro* fertilization program. *Horm. Res.*, **35**, 173–7

17. Belaisch-Allart, J.C., Hazout, A., Guillet-Rosso, F., Glissant, M., Testart, J. and Frydman, R. (1985). Various techniques for oocyte recovery in an *in*

vitro fertilization and embryo transfer program. *J. In Vitro Fertil. Embryo Transfer*, **2**, 99–104

18. Quigley, M.M. (1985). Selection of agents for enhanced follicular recruitment in an *in vitro* fertilization and embryo transfer replacement treatment program. *Ann. NY Acad. Sci.*, 442, 96–111

19. Belaisch-Allart, J., Dufetre, C., Allart, J.P. and Mouzon, J.D. (1991). Comparison of transvaginal and transabdominal ultrasound for monitoring follicular development in an *in vitro* fertilization programme. *Hum. Reprod.*, **6**, 688

20. Forman, R.G., Robinson, J., Yudkin, P., Egan, D., Reynolds, K. and Barlow, D.H. (1991). What is the true follicular diameter?: an assessment of the reproducibility of transvaginal ultrasound monitoring in stimulated cycles. *Fertil. Steril.*, **56**, 989–92

21. Fleischer, A.C., Herbert, C.M., Sacks, G.A., Wentz, A.C., Entman, S.S. and James Jr, A.E. (1986). Sonography of the endometrium during conception and non-conception cycles of *in vitro* fertilization and embryo transfer. *Fertil. Steril.*, **46**, 442–7

22. Welker, B.G., Gembruch, U., Diedrich, K., Al-Hasani, S. and Krebs, D. (1989). Transvaginal sonography of the endometrium during ovum pick-up in stimulated cycles for *in vitro* fertilization. *J. Ultrasound Med.*, **8**, 549–53

23. Gonen, Y. and Casper, R.F. (1990). Prediction of implantation by sonographic appearance of the endometrium during controlled ovarian stimulation for *in vitro* fertilization (IVF). *J. In Vitro Fertil. Embryo Transfer*, **7**, 146–52

24. Sher, G., Herbert, C., Maassarani, G. and Jacobs, M.H. (1991). Assessment of the late proliferative phase endometrium by ultrasonography in patients undergoing *in vitro* fertilization and embryo transfer (IVF/ET). *Hum. Reprod.* **6**, 232–7

25. Ueno, J., Oehninger, S., Brzyski, R.G., Acosta, A.A., Philput, C.B. and Muasher, S.J. (1991). Ultrasonographic appearance of the endometrium in natural and stimulated *in vitro* fertilization cycles and its correlation with outcome. *Hum. Reprod.*, **6**, 901–4

26. Khalifa, E., Brzyski, R.G., Oehninger, S., Acosta, A.A. and Muasher, S.J. (1992). Sonographic appearance of the endometrium: the predictive value for the outcome of *in vitro* fertilization in stimulated cycles. *Hum. Reprod.*, **7**, 677–80

27. Forman, R.G., Ross, C., Frydman, R., Egan, D. and Barow, D.H. (1990). Severe ovarian hyperstimulation syndrome using agonists of gonadotrophin releasing hormone for *in vitro* fertilization: a European series and a proposal for prevention. *Fertil. Steril.*, **53**, 502–9

28. Golan, A., Weinraub, Z., Ron-El, R., Soffer, Y., Herman, A. and Caspi, E. (1988). Ovarian hyperstimulation syndrome following D-Trp-6 luteinizing

hormone releasing hormone microcapsules and menotropin for *in vitro* fertilization. *Fertil. Steril.*, **50**, 912–16

29. MacDougall, M.J., Tan, S.L. and Jacobs, H.S. (1992). *In vitro* fertilization and the ovarian hyperstimulation syndrome. *Hum. Reprod.*, **7**, 597–600

30. Navot, D., Bergh, P.A. and Laufer, N. (1992). Ovarian hyperstimulation syndrome in novel reproductive technologies: prevention and treatment. *Fertil. Steril.*, **58**, 249–61

31. Blankstein, J., Shalev, J., Saadon, T., Kukia, E.E., Rabinovici, J., Pariente, C., Lunenfeld, B., Serr, D.M. and Maschiach, S. (1987). Ovarian hyperstimulation syndrome: prediction by number and size of preovulatory ovarian follicles. *Fertil. Steril.*, **47**, 597

5

Natural cycle *in vitro* fertilization: is there a place?

E.A. Lenton, A. Kumar, K. Turner, B.J. Woodward and I.D. Cooke

NATURAL CYCLE IVF: HISTORICAL PERSPECTIVE

The concept of collecting mature preovulatory human oocytes from the ovary, fertilizing them *in vitro* and transferring the resulting embryos back to the uterus was developed originally by Patrick Steptoe and Robert Edwards during the 1970s. Although their early attempts were fraught with difficulties their efforts were eventually successful and culminated in the birth of Louise Brown in 1978[1]. Encouraged by this success, a number of other groups attempted natural cycle *in vitro* fertilization (IVF) but were unable to produce pregnancies[2,3]. With hindsight it is easy to understand why natural cycle IVF should have been so difficult. Firstly, the assay systems available for detecting the luteinizing hormone (LH) surge were inaccurate, non-specific and slow. Knowledge of the characteristics of follicle growth and spontaneous ovulation were limited and egg recovery could only be achieved laparoscopically. The timing of egg collection, which we now know to be critical to within a few hours, was then largely a random phenomenon due to the inefficiencies of the hormone monitoring and the difficulties of organizing the operative procedures to take place at short notice, perhaps at night. Combining the data from the early reported studies, it can be calculated that only 58% of laparoscopies were successful in yielding one or more eggs and only 57% of these eggs were subsequently fertilized, probably because of the rather primitive methods available for preparing the sperm. A total of 72 embryos was transferred and these produced four clinical pregnancies (5.5% per embryo transfer) and two live births (2.8% per embryo transfer). Not surprisingly, natural cycle IVF was abandoned in favour of stimulated IVF purely because of the much greater probability of obtaining several eggs and embryos per patient.

During the late 1980s and early 1990s, in part as a reaction to the complexity, cost and appreciable hazards of stimulated IVF, the efficacy of natural cycle IVF was re-examined by a number of groups. Ranoux and colleagues[4] reported a pregnancy rate of 20% per embryo transfer in a series of 30 cycles, and this same group subsequently described a larger series of 80 cycles with a pregnancy rate of 32%[5]. Later, Svalander and colleagues reported a similar pregnancy rate of 30.8% in a series of 83 cycles[6]. Despite these encouraging data, other groups were unable to replicate their results. Paulson and co-workers[7] achieved a 13% pregnancy rate per embryo transfer in a series of 78 egg collections and concluded that it was reasonable to offer patients with tubal infertility up to three attempts at natural cycle IVF as an alternative to stimulated IVF. Claman and associates[8] considered that natural cycle IVF was an inefficient therapy for tubal infertility, in comparison with superovulation, because although they reported a pregnancy rate of 11% per embryo transfer, only 24% of the cycles they started reached embryo transfer. Most recently, a prospective randomized trial of natural versus clomiphene citrate-stimulated cycles failed to obtain any pregnancies in the natural cycle group, although it should be noted that 10 of 14 cycles were cancelled before egg collection because the spontaneous LH surge had started[9]. All these studies have a number of features in common. Firstly, the reported series were generally small, the largest describing only 83 cycles. Secondly, the patients were highly selected for tubal infertility (80–100%); male factor patients and women over 39 years were excluded. All of the groups were already operating stimulated IVF programmes and their expectations were to achieve comparable results using the natural cycle. Most had inadequate LH monitoring facilities (maximum of once per day), and even if LH was measured, the information was not used to time egg collection. For this purpose human chorionic gonadotrophin (hCG) was given according to standard protocols, and egg collection planned for 36 h later. Some groups cancelled patients if the spontaneous LH surge had begun before hCG was given, with the result that cancellation rates were unacceptably high. The combined outcome data for the early (1980–1982; refs. 1–3) series and

Table 1 Comparison of the efficiency of each stage of the *in vitro* fertilization (IVF) procedure in the early series of natural cycle IVF reports (refs. 1–3) and the more recently published reports (refs. 5–9)

	Early series (1980–1982)					Later series (1989–1994)				
Cycles started	216					343				
Eggs collected	126	**58%**				216	**63%**			
Embryos transferred	72	33%	**57%**			174	50%	**80%**		
Clinical pregnancies	4	2%	3%	**6%**		41	12%	19%	**24%**	
Live births	2	1%	2%	3%	**50%**	31	9%	14%	18%	**76%**

the later (1989–1994; refs. 5–9) series are shown in Table 1. The proportion of cycles started which resulted in successful egg collection did not improve significantly (58–63%) despite better endocrine monitoring, chiefly because of a tendency to cancel the cycles of patients starting an endogenous LH surge. The relative absence of male factor infertility and improved methods of sperm preparation are reflected in a much greater proportion of eggs being fertilized and transferred (80%, compared with 57% in the early studies). Clinical pregnancy rates per embryo were now acceptable at 24% (and better than multiple embryo transfers in some stimulated IVF programmes) but pregnancy losses were still problematical at 24%. Live birth rates per cycle started also improved, from 1 to 9% in the later series.

NATURAL CYCLE IVF: THE SHEFFIELD EXPERIENCE

Natural cycle IVF was commenced in Sheffield, UK in 1987. At that time a rapid urinary LH assay system was used and egg recovery was achieved via the transvesical–transabdominal route. Although pregnancies were achieved[10], the urinary endocrine monitoring employed was laborious and unreliable. Plasma sampling for LH was introduced in 1988, initially three times daily but decreasing to twice daily when rapid oestradiol assays became available in late 1989. Vaginal ultrasound-directed egg recoveries were introduced from 1989, and various other modifications to the natural cycle programme were also established as described by Lenton and colleagues[10]. Stimulated IVF was performed in parallel from 1989 onwards. The objectives of the natural cycle programme were multiple: firstly to establish optimum conditions for utilizing the natural cycle efficiently; secondly to describe the functional capacity of the spontaneously matured gametes in women with normal and abnormal reproductive function; and thirdly to compare and contrast embryo development and outcomes in women who progressed from natural to stimulated IVF treatment. Between 1987 and 1993, approximately 2400 attempts at natural cycle IVF were made and 110 pregnancies initiated. As with all IVF programmes, changes are introduced periodically, such as alterations to the culture medium[11], the methods of sperm preparation and other aspects of the procedures[12,13] and initially our relatively low natural cycle pregnancy rates were thought to be due in part to inefficiencies in the programme. However, when the results obtained over a 6-year period were examined, the improvement over time was relatively small (Table 2). Without any form of patient selection, live birth rates in years 5 and 6, when the programme was considered to be optimal, were only 12.2% per embryo transferred, compared with 8.1% in years 1 and 2 when the programme was in its infancy. Clinical pregnancy losses did decline steadily from 26% in 1988/89 to 14% in 1992/93, suggesting that at least some of the programme modifications had been of benefit.

One explanation for the relatively small improvement in pregnancy rates could have been the impact of patients returning for further attempts at natural cycle IVF. In this situation it is possible that the more fertile women will conceive early, leaving a progressively less fertile population attending for successive treatments. However, patients in our series never had more than two natural cycles of IVF with embryo transfer without being advised to change to an alternative form of treatment. Amongst those patients who did have two embryo-transfer cycles the probability of conception in the second cycle was only slightly lower than in the first (Table 3) and there was a small trend toward increased pregnancy loss following the second embryo transfer.

Table 2 Implantation, clinical pregnancy and live birth rates achieved between 1988 and 1993 using natural cycle *in vitro* fertilization. The data represent all embryos transferred, regardless of infertility indication or patient age. Implantation was defined as an human chorionic gonadotrophin (hCG) level >10 U/l and a clinical pregnancy as hCG >800 U/l, unless there was independent corroboration such as histological confirmation of an ectopic pregnancy, or ultrasound evidence of a gestation sac

	1988 + 1989	*1990 + 1991*	*1992 + 1993*
Embryos transferred	173	316	197
Rates per embryo transferred			
implantation (%)	13.9	13.6	18.8
clinical pregnancies (%)	11.0	12.7	14.2
live births (%)	8.1	10.1	12.2
clinical pregnancy losses (%)	26.3	20.0	14.3

The data cited above are expressed as clinical pregnancies and live births per embryo transfer, rather than per treatment cycle started. The reason for this is that a significant proportion of natural cycle IVF attempts fail to reach the embryo transfer stage and, if no embryo is available, there is clearly no possibility of pregnancy. Failure to recover or fertilize the single egg available in the spontaneous cycle is one of the major limitations of natural cycle IVF. There are at least seven critical stages between starting a cycle and ending with a live birth. None of these stages can be perfect, and cumulatively they will significantly reduce the overall efficiency of the system. For example, even with the most careful endocrine monitoring, a proportion of women will ovulate before the time set for egg collection, a proportion of follicles will rupture on needle entry (causing failure to collect an egg) and in a further number, no egg will be recovered despite systematic follicle flushing. Between January 1991 and December 1993, 676 cycles of natural cycle IVF were started in Sheffield; the losses at each stage are shown in Table 4. In this series, 82% of the natural cycles started resulted in successful egg collection. This is equivalent to a cancellation rate of 18%, which is relatively high in comparison to stimulated IVF with

Table 3 Implantation, clinical pregnancy and live birth rates following the first or second single embryo transfer (ET) resulting from all attempts at natural cycle IVF undertaken between 1991 and 1993

	First ET	*Second ET*
Embryos transferred	281	68
Rates per embryo transferred		
implantation (%)	18.5	20.6
clinical pregnancies (%)	16.0	14.7
live births (%)	13.5	11.8
clinical pregnancy losses (%)	15.6	20.0

its safety margin of multiple follicles. Similarly, collecting multiple eggs offers protection against occasional abnormal oocytes such as those with fragile zonae. If an egg is found to be abnormal in the natural cycle, the IVF attempt is automatically a failure. In our series only 91% of eggs collected were actually inseminated; the other 9% were considered to be damaged or abnormal. It is well known that not all eggs will fertilize normally – some may be polyspermic and others may not fertilize at all. Clearly, the proportion of male factor patients in an IVF programme will moderate this statistic. In this unselected series of patients, which included significant amounts of male factor infertility, only 72% of the cycles with normal eggs resulted in normal fertilization. Not all fertilized embryos will continue dividing normally; some may arrest, and so only 97% of the embryos formed in this series were actually replaced into the uterus. As with all IVF programmes, the most inefficient stage is when loss of replaced embryos occurs before implantation. Natural cycle IVF is no exception, with only 19% of this series of single embryo replacements resulting in maternal hCG levels greater than 10 U / l. Some embryos will be lost relatively early (biochemical pregnancy), but 83% will progress to become a recognized clinical pregnancy (defined here as a gestation sac on ultrasound and / or an hCG level > 800 U / l). Despite this, only a further 84% of these clinical pregnancies will continue, to result eventually in a live birth (Table 4). This represents an overall clinical pregnancy loss rate of 16%.

Table 4 The numbers of patients continuing from one stage to the next during natural cycle IVF treatment. The data represent all cycles started between January 1991 and December 1993, including those where donor sperm were used or the woman was over 40 years of age

Cycles started	676						
Eggs collected	553	**82%**					
Eggs inseminated	504	75%	**91%**				
Fertilized normally	361	54%	65%	**72%**			
Embryos transferred	349	53%	63%	69%	**97%**		
Implantations	66	10%	12%	13%	18%	**19%**	
Clinical pregnancies	55	8%	10%	11%	15%	16%	**83%**
Live births	46	7%	8%	9%	13%	13%	70%	**84%**

The overall efficiency of natural cycle IVF can be calculated as the product of each of these stages described above, i.e. $0.82 \times 0.91 \times 0.72 \times 0.97 \times 0.19 \times 0.83 \times 0.84$, to give a live birth rate per cycle started of 6.9%. Assuming that the efficiency of each of the stages could be improved by a small amount, the ultimate success rate that could theoretically be achieved using the technique can easily be calculated. For example, setting the efficiency of each stage at 90%, 95%, 85%, 98%, 25%, 90% and 90%, respectively, would still only give a live birth rate for natural cycle IVF of 14.4% per cycle started. This simple example illustrates effectively the point that no matter how well natural cycle IVF is performed, it will never result in adequate pregnancy rates unless embryos can be produced that each have a greater than 25% chance of implanting. At the present time, when considering the performance of gametes from infertile couples, this expectation seems remote. The occasional publications which have recorded pregnancy rates greater than those shown to be theoretically possible have probably been influenced by careful patient selection, or by the small numbers of cycles evaluated.

The critical or rate-limiting factor, as shown in Table 4, is the probability of implantation of the single embryo. In our series this was observed to be 19% for the single embryo resulting from each natural cycle attempt in a large unselected population of infertile couples. In a parallel series of multiple embryo replacements following stimulated egg collection (in a similar population of unselected infertile couples) the implantation rate per embryo (rather than per cycle with multiple embryo transfer) was identical (Table 5). Indeed, implantation and clinical pregnancy losses expressed on a per embryo basis were similar in both the natural cycle and the stimulated cycle series. Thus, live birth rates per embryo replaced were also identical at 13%, demonstrating that there is no real difference between natural and stimulated embryos. However, while the live birth rate per patient with embryo transfer remained at 13% in the natural cycle series, the stimulated IVF patients experienced a 23% live birth rate as a consequence of their multiple embryo transfers. There were no multiple pregnancies amongst the natural cycles, compared with 41% in the stimulated cycle series. Thus, although natural cycle IVF is capable of only low live birth rates per embryo transfer (13%) or per cycle started (7%), it does eliminate, at least in our hands, the risk of a multiple delivery.

NATURAL CYCLE IVF: THE CURRENT SITUATION

From information published by the Human Fertilisation and Embryology Authority it would appear that a number of other IVF clinics in the UK are practising natural cycle IVF and that several hundred cycles are performed annually. At the time of writing the latest outcome statistics available were those relating to the year 1992 and consisted of the annual returns from our centre as well as those from all other centres practising natural cycle IVF[14]. In order to allow a direct comparison between the results obtained by us during 1992 and those obtained by the other clinics in the UK, the published statistics were simply recalculated after subtraction of the 1992 Sheffield data, as shown in Table 6.

During 1992, 195 natural cycle IVF attempts were started in Sheffield, compared with an estimated 502 cycles for the rest of the UK. Whilst 89.2% of the Sheffield patients had eggs collected, only 56.3% of the

Table 5   Comparison of the ability of either natural cycle or stimulated *in vitro* fertilization (IVF) embryos to implant, develop to a recognized clinical pregnancy and finally to result in a live birth. The natural cycle data represent all cycles with embryos transferred between January 1991 and December 1993. The stimulated cycles are all cycles performed between January 1992 and December 1993 and the data are expressed on a per embryo basis, counting failed pregnancies as implantation of a single embryo only, unless two gestation sacs or foetal hearts were present. Other definitions are as described for Table 3

	Natural cycle IVF				*Stimulated IVF*			
Embryos transferred	349				1112			
Implantations	66	**19%**			208	**19%**		
Clinical pregnancies	55	16%	**83%**		185	17%	**89%**	
Live births	46	13%	70%	**84%**	139	13%	67%	**75%**

other UK cycles resulted in the collection of one or more eggs. Thus, in Sheffield the cycle cancellation rate was 10.9% while in the rest of the UK it was 43.6%. As a consequence, nearly double the Sheffield patients (65%) had an embryo replaced, compared with about 37% for the rest of the UK. The surprising aspect is that the embryos transferred in the rest of the UK cycles produced twice the clinical pregnancy rate per embryo transfer (22.3%) of the Sheffield embryo transfer cycles (11.1%). Consequently, any advantage gained by replacing embryos in many more cycles in Sheffield was lost because of the lower overall clinical pregnancy rate. Eventually, the live birth rates per cycle started were almost exactly the same (6.7 and 6.8% respectively) in the two series, despite the different technical and philosophical approaches. Interestingly, 20% of the UK natural cycle live births were recorded as being multiple, presumably twins, which is in direct contrast to our experience with completely unstimulated cycles.

Why should the live birth rate following natural cycle IVF remain at about 7% per cycle started, no matter how efficient the egg collection and embryo transfer stages? One possible explanation is that only a proportion of the eggs in any population of spontaneous cycles have the potential to produce embryos which can in turn implant and develop normally to term. Provided that the eggs 'with potential' are collected, fertilized and replaced, pregnancy yields will be optimized. Collection of additional eggs and embryos will not further increase the take-home baby rate. Thus, although we optimized the endocrine monitoring and the conditions of egg collection, such that we were able to collect eggs successfully from most patients (including those with poor quality or abnormal menstrual cycles), it seemed that the probability of conception was not increased compared with results from those groups which cancelled a much larger proportion of their natural cycles. During 1993 we decided to test this hypothesis by adopting a policy of cancelling, before egg collection, all cycles which were considered suboptimal – for example, those with an oestradiol peak of < 600 pmol/l, or where the follicular diameter was < 16 mm at the start of the LH surge. As expected, this policy had an immediate impact on our cancellation rates, which increased to 31.2% while the number of cycles which reached embryo transfer declined to 40.3% (Table 6). As with the 1992 UK data, the higher the cancellation rate, the greater the clinical pregnancy rate per embryo transfer cycle. In the 1993 Sheffield series, this rate reached 20.3% but, as predicted, there was no commensurate increase in live birth rates, which remained at 6.4%, similar to the 1992 series.

In principle, unselected population live birth rates of the order of 7% per cycle started are not considered high enough to justify an invasive procedure such as IVF, even though there are benefits, such as a minimal risk of multiple pregnancy and no associated hazard of ovarian hyper-stimulation. If, however, natural cycle IVF is attempted, high cancellation rates are considered desirable although more information is required on the specific characteristics of cycles which do not give rise to viable embryos. Utilizing a selective approach and collecting eggs only from the 'best' cycles should (theoretically) yield a good clinical pregnancy rate per embryo transfer, perhaps even approaching the predicted optimum of 25%. However, as a consequence of the deliberate cancellation of all inadequate cycles it would not then be meaningful to report pregnancy results in terms of 'cycles started', but rather as per 'embryos transferred', in order to permit comparability between patient types and between clinics.

The above analysis refers only to unselected patient populations, and it is possible that some patient subgroups will have a more acceptable outcome following natural cycle IVF than others. Alternatively, some patients who are known to respond poorly to stimulated IVF may not

Table 6 Comparison of the results of natural cycle *in vitro* fertilization (IVF) performed in Sheffield in 1992 and in the remainder of the UK in 1992. Data were obtained from the statistics published by the Human Fertilisation and Embryology Authority[14]. Also shown are the results of natural cycle IVF performed in Sheffield in 1993 when patients were selectively cancelled if their follicles developed abnormally. Cycles in which donor sperm were used have been excluded

	Sheffield *1992*	*Rest of UK* *1992*	*Sheffield* *1993*
Cycles started	195	502	157
Eggs collected	174	283	107
Embryos transferred	124	186	64
Clinical pregnancies	14	41	13
Live births	13	30	10
Cancellation rate (%)	10.9	43.6	31.8
Clinical pregnancy per embryo transfer (%)	11.3	22.0	20.3
Live births per embryo transfer (%)	10.4	16.1	15.6
Live births per cycle started (%)	6.7	6.8	6.4

have any worse outcome following natural cycle IVF. One such subgroup comprises the older women. It is well known that many older women do not respond well to ovarian stimulation, and even if they conceive following stimulated embryo transfer, there is a much increased risk of an early pregnancy loss. Analysis of two groups of women undergoing either natural or stimulated IVF in our clinic, during the same period of time, shows that the outcome of the natural cycle is far less influenced by maternal age than is the outcome of stimulated IVF (Table 7). In fact, live birth rates per cycle started are approximately constant at 6–7%, irrespective of age in the natural cycle, whereas there is a marked decline (from 24% to 6%) after stimulation between the younger and older women. Both treatments are associated with increasing pregnancy losses as the women become older, but these losses are more pronounced following stimulated IVF, so much so that in the 40+ years age-group, the two

Table 7 The effect of advancing maternal age on the pregnancy loss, live births per embryo transfer (ET) cycle and live births per cycle started, following natural cycle *in vitro* fertilization (IVF) (all cycles from January 1991 to December 1993) or stimulated IVF (all cycles from January 1992 to December 1993)

| | *Female age* (years) | | | |
	< 30	*30–34*	*35–39*	*≥ 40*
Natural cycle IVF				
Cycles started	137	305	185	48
Clinical pregnancies per ET (%)	14.3	16.5	15.0	19.0
Live births per cycle (%)	7.3	6.6	6.5	6.3
Stimulated IVF				
Cycles started	84	185	165	50
Clinical pregnancies per ET (%)	28.2	31.9	28.5	21.4
Live births per cycle (%)	22.6	23.4	18.2	6.0

treatments achieve comparable results. Clearly, the lower cost and greater simplicity of natural cycle IVF suggests that it may have a role in the treatment of the older woman, although the low live birth rates per cycle started still need to be justified in terms of treatment efficacy.

CONCLUSION

Natural cycle IVF is never likely to have a place in the widespread treatment of unselected infertile patient populations, as pregnancy rates per cycle will remain inadequately low. However, for selected subgroups of patients, such as the older woman, natural cycle IVF may offer outcomes that are equivalent to other forms of treatment, and so could be considered a viable alternative. IVF in the completely natural cycle, or following mild stimulation (e.g. clomiphene), may also have a valuable diagnostic role in assessing the capacity of the gametes to fertilize. Information gained in this way could then be used to inform further assisted conception treatment which could be as simple as ovarian stimulation and intrauterine insemination or, alternatively, could indicate the need for variations such as IVF in conjunction with intracytoplasmic sperm injection.

REFERENCES

1. Edwards, R.G., Steptoe, P.C. and Purdy, J.M. (1980). Establishing full-term human pregnancies using cleaving embryos grown *in vitro*. *Br. J. Obstet. Gynaecol.*, **87**, 737–56
2. Johnston, I., Lopata, A., Spiers, A., Hoult, I., Kellow, G. and du Plessis, Y. (1981). *In vitro* fertilisation: the challenge of the eighties. *Fertil. Steril.*, **36**, 699–706
3. Jones, H.W., Jones, G., Andrews, M.C., Acosta, A., Bundren, C., Garcia, J., Sandow, B., Veeck, L., Wilkes, C., Witmyer, J., Wortham, J.E. and Wright, G. (1982). The programme for *in vitro* fertilisation at Norfolk. *Fertil. Steril.*, **38**,14–21
4. Ranoux, C., Foulot, H., Dubuisson, J.B., Rambaud, D., Aubriot, F.-X. and Poirot, C. (1988). Returning to spontaneous cycles in *in vitro* fertilisation. *J. IVF and Embryo Transfer*, **5**, 304
5. Foulot, H., Ranoux, C., Dubuisson, J.B., Rambaud, D., Aubriot, F.-X. and Poirot, C. (1989). *In vitro* fertilisation without ovarian stimulation: a simplified protocol applied in 80 cycles. *Fertil. Steril.*, **52**, 617–21
6. Svalander, P., Green, B., Haglund, K., Hagstrom, B., Lindstedt, J.A., Marsk, L., Nygre, K.-G., Stefensson, M., Tocksberg, K. and Thornblad, A.-M. (1991). Natural versus stimulated IVF treatment for tubal factor infertility. *Hum. Reprod.*, **6**, (Suppl. 1), 101
7. Paulson, R.J., Sauer, M.V., Francis, M.M., Macaso, T.M. and Lobo, R.A. (1992). *In vitro* fertilisation in unstimulated cycles: the University of Southern California experience. *Fertil. Steril.*, **57**, 290–3
8. Claman, P., Domingo, M., Garner, P., Leader, A. and Spence, J.E.H. (1993). Natural cycle *in vitro* fertilisation–embryo transfer at the University of Ottawa: an inefficient therapy for tubal infertility. *Fertil. Steril.*, **60**, 298–302
9. MacDougall, M.J., Tan, S.-L., Hall, V., Balen, A., Mason, B.A. and Jacobs, H.S. (1994). Comparison of natural cycle IVF with clomiphene citrate-stimulated cycles in *in vitro* fertilisation: a prospective randomized trial. *Fertil. Steril.*, **61**,1052–7
10. Lenton, E.A., Cooke, I.D., Hooper, M., King, H., Kumar, A., Monks, N., Turner, K. and Verma, S. (1992). *In vitro* fertilisation in the natural cycle. *Clin. Obstet. Gynecol.*, **6**, 229–45

11. Monks, N.J., Turner, K., Hooper, M.A.K., Kumar, A., Verma, S. and Lenton, E.A. (1993). Development of embryos from natural cycle *in-vitro* fertilisation: impact of medium type and female infertility factors. *Hum. Reprod.*, **8**, 266–71

12. Ramsewak, S.S., Kumar, A., Welsby, R., Mowforth, A. and Lenton, E.A. (1990). Is analgesia required for transvaginal simple-follicle aspiration in *in vitro* fertilisation? A double blind study. *J. IVF and Embryo Transfer*, **7**, 299–305

13. Ramsewak, S.S., Cooke, I.D., Li, T.C., Kumar, A., Monks, N.J. and Lenton, E.A. (1990). Are factors that influence oocyte fertilisation also predictive? An assessment of 148 cycles of *in vitro* fertilisation without gonadotrophin stimulation. *Fertil. Steril.*, **54**, 470–4

14. Human Fertilisation and Embryology Authority. (1994). *Third Annual Report*, Annex 7, Table 2B, p.52. (London: HFEA)

6

Doppler ultrasound: a new refinement for *in vitro* fertilization

R.K. Goswamy

INTRODUCTION

In previous publications we have reported that uterine response to endogenous hormonal changes in spontaneous ovarian cycles can be demonstrated using Doppler ultrasound techniques[1]. These demonstrated that uterine perfusion increases in response to rising oestrogen levels during the follicular phase, decreases in the preovulatory phase in response to the preovulatory oestrogen fall, and increases in the luteal phase in response to the combined effect of oestrogen and progesterone.

We also reported that, in conception cycles, uterine perfusion continues to increase in the late luteal phase, in contrast to non-conception cycles where there is a premenstrual decrease in perfusion as a result of falling progesterone levels. Thus, it was postulated that Doppler ultrasound techniques could potentially be used to diagnose pregnancy prior to the date of expected onset of menses.

In a further study[2] we used the methodology previously devised to study the uterine perfusion response in those patients who had failed to conceive despite repeated multiple embryo replacement in *in vitro* fertilization (IVF) cycles. These patients, when studied during spontaneous ovarian cycles, had normal endocrine changes and endometrial thickness on ultrasound, and basal body temperature changes compatible with ovulatory cycles, but had an inadequate uterine perfusion response in 50% of the patients recruited to the study.

73

This chapter reports on a larger number of patients in this ongoing prospective study and describes a new quantitative method to measure uterine perfusion which will be shown to be superior to the conventional formulae used in flow velocity waveform analyses of Doppler ultrasound examinations.

PATIENTS AND METHODS

At the time of writing, 254 patients had been recruited for study. Recruitment was on the basis that three previous IVF attempts had been unsuccessful in achieving pregnancy, despite good gamete quality, in patients under the age of 40 years, although patients over this age were included if two previous such attempts had been unsuccessful.

Our criteria for assessing gamete quality have been described previously[3,4]. Briefly, if mean urinary LH levels were below 0.20 IU/l and over 60% of all the oocytes recovered were fertilized by the sperm, then we presumed that gamete quality was satisfactory.

In the initial 2½ years of the study, Doppler ultrasound studies were performed using a Philips SDD 600 spectrum analyser with a 3 MHz Doppler transducer which was offset on a 3.5 MHz imaging transducer attached to a Philips SDR 1550 imaging system (Philips Ultrasound Inc., California, USA). Scans were performed abdominally with the patient's bladder full enough to visualize the pulsations of the ascending branch of the uterine artery. The Doppler gate was placed over this area to obtain the typical uterine artery waveform as previously described by Taylor and colleagues[5]. In the latter part of the study Doppler ultrasound studies were performed using a 7.5 MHz vaginal imaging transducer, attached to the Siemens SL2 ultrasound machine with built-in 3 MHz Doppler crystals to obtain flow velocity waveforms from the ascending branch of the uterine artery in the oblique longitudinal plane.

The shape of the flow velocity waveform was similar to that obtained with the abdominal route. All studies were performed during spontaneous ovarian cycles and the waveform classification, modified resistance index and modified systolic/diastolic (S/D) ratio previously described were noted.

A new computer program using an Appleton Floscan system was used to devise another index, where the area under the systolic component of the flow velocity waveform (*S) was divided by the area under the diastolic component (*D). We have called this ratio (*S/*D) the 'Perfusion Index' (PeI). However, until adequate numbers of patients were recruited into the study to analyse the PeI, we continued to classify waveforms as Type O, A, B and C as previously described[1]. Type O and Type A waveforms obtained in the mid-secretory phase were taken to indicate decreased perfusion of the uterine vascular bed, and Type B or Type C waveforms were assumed to indicate good uterine perfusion.

Patients with good uterine perfusion (Type B or C) were designated Group I patients and those with poor uterine perfusion were allocated to Group II. Group I patients were advised to proceed with another IVF attempt with ovarian stimulation, as in previous attempts. Group II patients were prescribed tablets (Cyclo-Progynova® 2 mg, containing oestradiol valerate, 2 mg × 11 days and oestradiol valerate 2 mg and Norgesterel® 0.5 mg × 10 days (Schering Pharmaceutical Ltd., UK), to be taken for 21 days each cycle starting on the 5th day of menstruation.

Repeat Doppler studies were then performed after the patients had been on this treatment for 3 months. Patients with mid-secretory waveforms Type B or C were now considered to have satisfactory perfusion and advised to attempt IVF once again. In Group II patients, ovarian stimulation was carried out as before and the patients continued to take the oestradiol valerate tablets, 2 mg, throughout the follicular and luteal phases.

Patients exhibiting Type O or A waveforms, despite cyclical Cyclo-Progynova, were allocated to a third group, designated Group IIa. These patients underwent ovarian stimulation, oocyte recovery and IVF and the resulting embryos were cryopreserved. Further therapy followed, using rising doses of oestradiol valerate until good Doppler waveforms were observed (Type B or C) and, after progesterone supplementation, thawed embryos were replaced *in utero*.

Pregnancy rates of patients in Group I, II, IIa and 'first attemptors' were compared using χ^2 analyses, as were the pregnancy rates between Groups I, II, IIa and women who had previously had four or more attempts at pregnancy.

RESULTS

A total of 254 women was recruited onto the study at the time of this analysis, and 197 (77.5%) of these patients had completed hormone

Table 1 Waveform classification compared to Perfusion Index (PeI) in 187 flow velocity waveforms

Classification	*Perfusion Index* (mean ± SD)
Type A ($n = 65$)	3.11 ± 0.87 [*][†]
Type B ($n = 46$)	1.98 ± 0.58 [*]
Type C ($n = 76$)	1.81 ± 0.50 [†]

[*]Type A vs. Type B, $p < 0.001$; [†]Type A vs. Type C, $p < 0.001$; Type B vs. Type C, $p = 0.12$ (NS)

therapy and another IVF attempt. The results of these 187 treatment cycles are presented here.

The PeI was available for 187 flow velocity waveforms and its correlation with the waveform classification is shown in Table 1. Using χ^2 analysis, the mean PeI was highly significant between Type A and Type B waveforms ($p < 0.001$) and between Type A and Type C waveforms ($p < 0.001$). There was no significant difference between Type B and Type C waveforms ($p = 0.12$). Group I consisted of 107 (54.3%) women and Group II and IIa consisted of 90 (45.7%) patients. Nine (10%) of the 90 patients were allocated subsequently to Group IIa and underwent high-dose hormone therapy as described above.

Patients in Group I were treated with IVF therapy using the same ovarian stimulation as in previous attempts. A total of 107 of these patients had completed therapy at the time of analysis.

Patients in Group II were treated with cyclical hormone therapy, using tablets of Cyclo-Progynova as previously described, and Doppler studies were performed to assess uterine response in the mid-secretory phase. Of the 90 patients who had completed hormone therapy for a preliminary analysis, 58 (64%) achieved a Type C response, and 22 (24%) achieved a Type B response. Ten women (11%) failed to achieve an adequate uterine response with low-dose therapy and were allocated to Group IIa. Patients in Group IIa were treated with rising doses of oestrogen therapy in combination with progesterone therapy, as in those cases treated for donor oocytes[2]. The results of subsequent IVF therapy for patients in Group II

Table 2 Comparison of subsequent IVF therapy in Group I, II, and IIa patients with 'first attemptors'

	Number of patients	Number of pregnancies	Pregnancy rate (%)
First attempt	1828	429	26.9
Group I	107	31	28.97
Group II and IIa	90	24	26.67

p = NS for first attempt vs. Group I, or first attempt vs. Groups II and IIa

and Group IIa are shown together because the number of patients in Group IIa is too small for meaningful statistical analysis, but it has to be appreciated that they may represent different subgroups.

Table 2 shows the results of subsequent IVF therapy of patients in Group I and Group II. The pregnancy rate in these groups is compared with first attemptors, using χ^2 analyses. There was no significant difference in the pregnancy rate between any of these groups.

Table 3 compares the outcome of subsequent IVF therapy in Group I and II with patients who had four or more previous embryo replacements. There was a highly significant difference between the pregnancy rate achieved by Group I women and 'fourth attemptors' ($p < 0.001$) and a significant difference when the latter was compared to Group II patients ($p < 0.02$).

Of the ten patients in Group IIa, three (30%) achieved pregnancy with frozen–thawed embryos being replaced in cycles with rising doses of oestrogen and progesterone therapy.

DISCUSSION

This chapter has assessed uterine perfusion in women who have failed to achieve pregnancy despite repeated IVF attempts. In addition to confirming findings in previous publications, it also presents two additional methods to improve the use of this investigation in the management of infertile women.

Table 3 Comparison of subsequent IVF therapy in Group I, II and IIa patients with women who had had four or more attempts at pregnancy

	Number of patients	Number of pregnancies	Pregnancy rate (%)
Four or more attempts	316	54	17.4
Group I	107	31	28.97
Group II and IIa	90	24	26.67

$p < 0.001$ for Group I vs. four or more attempts; $p < 0.021$ for Group II vs. four or more attempts

Firstly, by using vaginal ultrasound techniques, patients can be scanned with an empty bladder. Not only more comfortable for patients, this method also increases the accuracy of waveform analysis. I have described the effect of an excessively full bladder causing a false-positive diagnosis of increased uterine resistance, such that Type A waveforms may be converted to Type B or C waveforms by asking the patient to partially void the urinary bladder. This can be obviated easily with the use of vaginal ultrasound examinations.

Secondly, the use of the Perfusion Index, or PeI, indicates a significant difference between Type A and Type B waveforms. In a previous publication[2], there was no significant difference between the modified resistance index or the modified S/D ratio, when these were used to differentiate between Type A and Type B waveforms. By such differentiation, it is now possible to numerically separate the patients with poor perfusion from those with a good uterine perfusion response.

Finally, the hypothesis which states that decreased uterine perfusion is a cause of infertility is closer to being proved by the results from this ongoing study. If poor uterine perfusion is a cause of failed implantation in IVF patients, then the fall in pregnancy rates associated with fourth or subsequent attempts may be attributed to this. That is, if patients with good uterine perfusion are allowed to go ahead with another IVF attempt, their pregnancy rate should be the same as first, second or third attemptors. The converse would apply if patients with poor uterine perfusion were allowed to go ahead without any hormone therapy prior to another IVF attempt. However, the provision of hormone therapy does improve uterine perfusion in these patients and the pregnancy rate in subsequent attempts does improve significantly. One could therefore conclude that decreased uterine perfusion is a cause of failed implantation. This would confirm that this is a cause of infertility hitherto unproven.

Why the uterus does not respond adequately to endogenous hormone changes in spontaneous cycle is unknown. I would postulate that there may be a degree of desensitization of receptors in the uterus to endogenous hormones which appear to control the mechanisms that increase uterine perfusion, thereby decreasing implantation and hence pregnancy rates.

If the mean pregnancy rate after the first three IVF attempts is 25%, then in an arbitrary group of 100 women, 40 would not be pregnant after three attempts. Our data would suggest that half of these would have poor uterine perfusion – i.e. 20% of all women undergoing IVF therapy! If other data substantiate these findings, it would give strength to the suggestion that all patients should have uterine artery Doppler flow studies, perhaps even before their first attempt at IVF. In this manner potential repeat failures might be selected out for interventive treatment at an early stage, hence increasing the overall success rate of IVF per cycle started.

REFERENCES

1. Goswamy, R.K. and Steptoe, P.C. (1988). Doppler ultrasound studies of the uterine artery in spontaneous ovarian cycles. *Hum. Reprod.*, **3**, 721–6
2. Goswamy, R.K., Williams, G. and Steptoe, P.C. (1988). Decreased uterine perfusion – a cause of infertility. *Hum. Reprod.*, **3**, 955–9
3. Howles, C.M., Macnamee, M., Edwards, R.G., Goswamy, R.K. and Steptoe, P.C. (1986). The effect of high tonic levels of luteinizing hormone on outcome of *in vitro* fertilization. *Lancet*, **2**, 521–2
4. Steptoe, P.C., Edwards, R.G. and Walters, D.E. (1986). Observations on 767 clinical pregnancies and 500 births after *in vitro* fertilization. *Hum. Reprod.*, **1**, 89–94
5. Taylor, K.J.W., Burns, P.N., Wells, P.N.T., Conway, D.I. and Hull, M.G.R. (1985). Ultrasound Doppler flow studies of the ovarian and uterine arteries. *Br. Med. Obstet. Gynaecol.*, **92**, 240–6

7

Recombinant human follicle stimulating hormone

B. A. Lieberman⋆

INTRODUCTION

Follicle stimulating hormone (FSH), one of two gonadotrophin hormones secreted by the pituitary gland, regulates the growth of the Graafian follicle in the female. This is accomplished via membrane receptors in the granulosa cells causing adenylate cyclase activation. The granulosa cells synthesize oestrogens and secrete other ovarian factors essential for cell differentiation and gamete maturation[1,2].

The α and β subunits of FSH are glycoproteins; the α chain has 92 amino acids and the β, 111. Each subunit has two complex heterogeneous N-linked oligosaccharide chains. Variations in the glycosylation results in a spectrum of isoforms with differences in net charge bioactivities and elimination half-life[3].

More than 30 years have elapsed since the introduction of urinary-derived human menopausal gonadotrophin (hMG) for the treatment of anovulation[4]. The production of hMG requires the collection of vast quantities of urine from groups of menopausal women. The difficulties associated with this collection, and of contamination with other urinary

⋆The work described in this chapter was carried out in a number of centres and is presented on behalf of the European Puregon® Study Group and the Section of Reproductive Medicine and Biometrics Medical Research and Development Unit, NV Organon, Oss, Holland

81

excreted hormones (e.g. chorionic gonadotrophin) and purification, necessitated the development of recombinant human FSH (rhFSH, Puregon®, Organon). The rhFSH is 99% pure, whilst the active substance in urinary-derived FSH (uFSH) has a limited biochemical purity (1–3% w/w).

The expression of human FSH in Chinese hamster ovary (CHO) cells transfected with both subunit genes[5,6] resulted in the synthesis of human FSH. The polypeptide backbone of rhFSH is indistinguishable from that of natural FSH, whereas recombinant and natural carbohydrate chain structures are closely related[7]. The small structural difference does not affect charge heterogeneity, receptor-binding affinity or *in vitro* and *in vivo* bioactivity of rhFSH[8,9].

To date, clinical studies have suggested that the use of rhFSH is safe and without adverse effects. Studies in gonadotrophin-deficient volunteers have demonstrated that the elimination half-life of serum FSH after intramuscular injection of rhFSH or uFSH (Metrodin®) is similar[10–13]. In a pilot study, rhFSH was shown to be both safe and effective for controlled ovarian hyperstimulation, in conjunction with different GnRH agonist regimens[14].

AIM AND STUDY DESIGN

The aim of the study was to determine the safety and effectiveness of rhFSH after pituitary desensitization with a luteinizing hormone releasing hormone (LHRH) analogue (buserelin, Suprefact®, Hoechst) in infertile women being treated by *in vitro* fertilization, by comparison to a similar but urinary-derived FSH preparation (uFSH, urofollitrophin, Metrodin®, Serono). This prospective, randomized, assessor-blind trial was undertaken at 18 European clinics between March 1993 and August 1994 by members of the European Puregon Study Group.

PATIENTS AND METHODS

Prior to the commencement of the study, standardized protocols for drug administration and assessment of oocyte maturity and embryo quality were agreed. The only permissible differences in therapy related to the

Table 1 Embryo quality

Type	Description
1	All blastomeres have an equal size without the presence of anucleate fragments
2	Not all blastomeres have an equal size; anucleate fragments present in less than 20% of volume
3	Not all blastomeres have an equal size; anucleate fragments present in more than 20% volume
4	The embryo is totally fragmented

dose at which the FSH was commenced and the drugs used to support the luteal phase. The main measures of outcome were the total number of oocytes recovered and the clinical pregnancy rate per cycle.

Other measures included the number of follicles $\geq$ 15 and 17 mm, the serum FSH and oestradiol concentrations on the day of human chorionic gonadotrophin (hCG) administration, the total number of FSH ampoules used, the duration of FSH administration, the number of mature oocytes collected, the sum of type 1 and 2 embryos (Table 1) and the implantation rate. The criteria for inclusion and patient selection were:

(1) Women ranging in age from 18–39 years at the time of screening.

(2) Cause of infertility potentially treatable by *in vitro* fertilization (IVF).

(3) A maximum of three previous IVF, gamete (GIFT) or zygote (ZIFT) intrafallopian transfer attempts in which oocytes were collected at least once.

(4) Normal ovulatory cycles with a mean length ranging between 24 and 35 days and an intra-individual variation of plus or minus 3 days (but never outside the 24–35 days range).

(5) Sound physical and mental health.

(6) Body weight between 80 and 130% of the ideal body weight.

(7) Able to give written informed consent.

Women or couples showing any of the following were ineligible for entry in the trial:

(1) Infertility caused by endocrine abnormalities including hyperprolactinaemia, polycystic ovary syndrome and absence of ovarian function.

(2) Male infertility defined by the following critera: $< 10 \times 10^6$ sperm per ml and/or $< 40\%$ normal morphology and/or $< 40\%$ normal motility.

(3) Contraindications for the use of gonadotrophin releasing hormone (GnRH) analogues, FSH, hMG, and/or hCG.

(4) Any ovarian and/or abdominal abnormality that would interfere with adequate ultrasound investigation.

(5) Hypertension (sitting diastolic blood pressure > 90 mmHg and/or systolic blood pressure > 150 mmHg).

(6) Chronic cardiovascular, hepatic, renal or pulmonary disease.

(7) History of (within 12 months) or current abuse of alcohol or drugs.

(8) Administration of investigational drugs within 3 months prior to screening.

Pituitary desensitization using buserelin by nasal sniffing, 4×150 µg/day was commenced on the first day of menses. The buserelin could be continued for a maximum of 4 weeks. Complete desensitization was confirmed by serum oestradiol < 50 pg/ml, 2 weeks after commencement of the drug. Cystic lesions in the ovary (> 10 mm) were treated by aspiration and/or extension of the buserelin for an additional 2 weeks.

Follicular stimulation using either 150 or 225 IU FSH by intramuscular injection for 4 days was commenced once pituitary desensitization had been achieved. The dose of FSH was adjusted thereafter, according to individual requirements or clinic protocols. Ovulation was initiated by 10 000 IU hCG when three or more follicles measured 17 mm in diameter. Oocyte recovery was performed invariably using a vaginal ultrasound probe 35 h after the hCG injection. A maximum of three early cleavage embryos were replaced transvaginally 48–72 h after oocyte recovery.

Luteal phase support varied according to clinic practice, ranging from three injections of 1500 IU hCG to progesterone 50 mg (intramuscularly) or 400 mg (per vaginum) per day.

STATISTICAL METHODS

For ordinal data, analyses of variance (ANOVA) were performed and, if not applicable, the Wilcoxon test statistic, adjusting for centre or, equivalently, the Mantel–Haenszel test statistic extended for multiple centres using standardized mid-rank scores per centre. A parametric analysis based on Cochran[15] and Whitehead's[16] methods of combining individual centre results was applied and used for communication of results and eventual analysis, next to the Wilcoxon results. Analyses of covariance (ANCOVA) techniques were performed to investigate the influence of prognostic factors on the treatment comparisons. For binary data, the Mantel–Haenszel test statistic extended for multiple centres was used to logistic regression for consolidation of these results and as means of performing analyses incorporating prognostic factors.

RESULTS

A total of 1027 women were randomly allocated in a ratio of 3:2, with regard to follicular stimulation using either rhFSH or uFSH. Their demographic details and infertility profiles are shown in Table 2.

Cycle cancellations

The outcome of the randomization process is shown in Table 3. A total of 152 subjects started FSH treatment but did not have an embryo transfer (rhFSH: $n = 85$, 14.5%; uFSH: $n = 67$, 16.9%; not significantly different). A low response was reported in 27 subjects in the rhFSH group (32%) and in 30 of the uFSH group (45%). Risk of ovarian hyperstimulation was the reason for cancellation in 12 rhFSH-treated subjects (14%) and six uFSH-treated subjects (9%). In 29 subjects (34%) failed fertilization was the reason for discontinuation in the rhFSH group, compared to 16 (24%) in the urinary FSH group.

Table 2 Demographic and infertility characteristics. rhFSH, recombinant human FSH; uFSH, urinary-derived FSH

Characteristic	*rhFSH*	*uFSH*
Mean age (years)	32.2	32.3
Mean weight (kg)	61.3	61.2
Mean height (cm)	164.4	164.3
Number (%) of subjects with cause of infertility:		
tubal disease	377 (64.4)	254 (64.1)
endometriosis	45 (7.7)	30 (7.6)
tubal disease + endometriosis	23 (3.9)	15 (3.8)
unknown	117 (20.0)	79 (19.9)
other	23 (4.0)	18 (4.5)
Mean duration of infertility (years)	6.3	6.1
Number (%) of subjects with primary infertility	259 (44.3)	174 (43.9)
Number (%) of subjects with secondary infertility	326 (55.7)	222 (56.1)

The biological response to the drugs administered is shown in Table 4. The use of rhFSH was also associated with significantly more follicles of > 15 mm diameter, higher oestradiol concentrations and lower FSH levels on the day of hCG. Significantly less rhFSH was used to achieve the required number and size of follicles prior to the hCG. (Table 4).

Outcome of treatment

The outcome of treatment is shown in Table 5. Significantly more oocytes and a significantly higher number of mature oocytes were recovered after follicular stimulation with rhFSH.

More grade 1 and 2 embryos developed after stimulation with rhFSH than with uFSH but there was no difference in the implantation rate nor in the number of women who conceived after treatment with either drug.

Table 3 Outcome of randomization. rhFSH, recombinant human FSH; uFSH, urinary-derived FSH

Category	rhFSH	uFSH	Total
Number of women to receive	615	412	1027
Number of women commencing buserelin	602	405	1007
Number of cycles of embryo replacement	500	329	829

Safety

No differences were observed with respect to the number or severity of drug-related side-effects or complications.

The ovarian hyperstimulation syndrome leading to hospitalization was seen in 19 of 585 rhFSH-treated subjects (3.2%) and in eight of the 396 uFSH-treated subjects (2.0%; not significantly different). In 545 rhFSH-treated and 353 uFSH-treated subjects spare serum samples could be assessed for the presence of anti-FSH and anti-CHO cell-derived protein antibodies. No relevant antibody concentrations were found.

No clinically relevant changes from baseline of routine blood biochemistry, haematology and urinalysis were detected.

DISCUSSION

The data reported in this paper were first published in 1994 and encompass the largest prospective comparative drug trial in infertile human females treated by IVF after pituitary desensitization with an LHRH analogue and follicular stimulation using either rhFSH or a similar but urinary-derived preparation urofollitrophin[17].

The rhFSH was biologically more effective, as less drug was required to reach the criteria for the injection of hCG; more oocytes were recovered and their quality, and that of the embryos replaced, was improved. This notion of enhanced bioactivity was not anticipated but is shown by the recruitment of more follicles, higher oestradiol concentrations and

Table 4 Biological response to stimulation. rhFSH, recombinant human FSH; uFSH, urinary-derived FSH; hCG, human chorionic gonadotrophin

	Mean (adjusted for centre)		*Recombinant minus uFSH*	
Parameter	*rhFSH*	*uFSH*	*Difference*	*95% CI*★
Number of follicles > 15 mm on day of hCG	7.49	6.67	0.81	0.4–1.2 ($p < 0.0001$)
Number of follicles > 17 mm on day of hCG	4.61	4.38	0.23	-0.0–0.5 ($p = 0.09$)
Maximum serum oestradiol (pmol/l)	6084	5179	905	494–1317 ($p < 0.0001$)
Serum FSH on day of hCG (IU/l)	11.5	12.1	-0.6	-1.1–-0.1 ($p = 0.03$)
Total number of ampoules used	28.5	31.8	-3.3	-4.5–-2.1 ($p < 0.0001$)
Treatment length (days)	10.7	11.3	-0.6	-0.9–-0.3 ($p < 0.0001$)
Number of mature oocytes recovered	8.6	6.8	1.8	1.1–2.4 ($p < 0.0001$)
Number of good-quality embryos	3.1	2.6	0.5	0.2–0.8 ($p = 0.003$)

★CI = confidence interval

reduced FSH levels on the day of hCG injection, and the reduced amount of rhFSH required to achieve satisfactory follicular growth prior to oocyte recovery. However, this does not result in higher rates of implantation nor pregnancy after the replacement of a maximum of three fresh early-cleavage embryos. These measures may be too crude to reflect this effect, in view of the large number of variables which influence implantation and pregnancy outcome. The enhanced bioactivity may possibly be reflected in the outcome of the cryopreserved embryos generated in the original study. These data are not yet available.

These results may also be interpreted as a reduction in the bioactivity of uFSH, rather than as an enhanced activity of rhFSH possibly due to

Table 5 Outcome of treatment. rhFSH, recombinant human FSH; uFSH, urinary-derived FSH

Parameter	Mean (adjusted for centre)		Recombinant minus uFSH	
	rhFSH	*uFSH*	*Difference*	*95% CI**
Implantation rate (%)	0.11	0.09	0.01	-0.02–0.05 ($p = 0.40$)
Clinical pregnancy rate (%) per attempt	29.3	25.3	4.0	-1.6–9.6 ($p = 0.17$)
Clinical pregnancy rate (%) per transfer	34.3	30.5	3.8	-2.6–10.3 ($p = 0.25$)

*CI = confidence interval

contamination with other urinary protein fractions, or to less active substance in each international unit of uFSH. Robertson has demonstrated the batch-to-batch variation of LH/hCG in Pergonal®, but no significant variability was present within each batch[18]. The drugs used in this study were standardized according to the European Pharmacopoeia[19]. Should further studies confirm the significant difference in bioactivity between 75 IU rhFSH and ostensibly the same amount of uFSH, further consideration of the standard and reference protocols will be necessary[20].

It is debatable whether the introduction of recombinant human FSH represents a major advance in the management of anovulatory women, and to stimulate the development of multiple follicles prior to treatment by IVF and other assisted reproductive techniques. On the positive side, the drug may be self-administered as a subcutaneous injection and it is now the drug of choice in those women who exhibit allergic phenomena after intramuscular injections with human menopausal gonadotrophin. The cost of rhFSH and the continued availability and price of hMG will to a large extent determine its place in the market. Should the results of this study be confirmed, and if an improvement in the cumulative pregnancy rate per cycle of stimulation associated with the replacement of the extra freeze–thawed embryos become a reality, an additional role for rhFSH will be apparent.

SUMMARY

The results of a prospective multicentre study indicate that recombinant human follicle stimulating hormone (rhFSH) is as safe as FSH derived from urine (uFSH, urofollitrophin, Metrodin®, Serono) for ovarian stimulation in infertile women after pituitary desensitization prior to treatment by *in vitro* fertilization. The rhFSH was biologically more potent, requiring less drug to achieve satisfactory follicular growth prior to oocyte recovery. The enhanced bioactivity was associated with increased oocyte recruitment and improved oocyte and embryo quality, but no difference in the pregnancy rate was apparent after the replacement of up to three fresh embryos. The outcome of treatment with the replacement of freeze–thawed embryos has yet to be determined.

ACKNOWLEDGEMENTS

This chapter was written on behalf of the European Puregon® Study Group, whose members are: P. Devroey (Brussels), P. Hornnes (Copenhagen), K. Diedrich (Bonn), L. Wildt (Erlangen), P. Barri (Barcelona), R. Forman (London), B. Lieberman (Manchester), R. Shaw (Cardiff), C. West (Edinburgh), R. Winston (London), B. Tarlatzis (Thessaloniki), Z. Shoham (Rehovot), R. Harrison (Dublin), T. Abyholm (Oslo), J. Khan (Trondheim), A. Tiitinen (Helsinki), L. Hamberger (Goteborg) and N. Sjoberg (Malmo), and also of the Section of Reproductive Medicine and Biometrics, Medical Research and Development Unit, NV Organon, Oss, The Netherlands: H.J. Out, B.M.J.L. Mannaerts, H.J.T. Coelingh Bennink and S.G.A.J. Driessen.

REFERENCES

1. Hsueh, A.J., Adashi, E.Y., Jones, P.B. and Welsh, T.H. (1984). Hormonal regulation of the differentiation of cultured ovarian granulosa cells. *Endocr. Rev.*, **5**, 76–127

2. Sharp, R.M. (1990). Intratesticular control of steroidogenesis. *Clin. Endocrinol.*, **33**, 787–97

3. Boime, I., Keene, J., Galway, A.B., Fares, F.A., LaPolt, P. and Hseuh, A.J. (1990). Expression of recombinant human FSH, LH and hCG

in mammalian cells: a model for probing functional determinants. In Hunzicker-Dunn, M. and Schwartz, N.B., (eds.) *Follicle Stimulating Hormone: Regulation of Secretion and Molecular Mechanisms of Action*, pp. 120–8 (Norwell M A: Serono Symposia USA)

4. Lunenfeld, B. and Insler, V. (1990). Induction of ovulation: historical aspects. *Baillière's Clin. Obstet. Gynaecol.*, **4**, 473–89

5. Van Wezenbeek, P., Draaier, J., Van Meel, F. and Olijve, W. (1990). Recombinant follicle stimulating hormone I. Construction, selection and characterization of a cell line. In Crommelin, D.J.A. and Schellekens, H.(eds.) *From Clone to Clinic, Developments in Biotherapy*, pp. 245–51 (New York: Kluwer)

6. Keene, J.L., Matzuk, M.M., Otani, T., Fauser, B.C., Galway, A.B., Hsueh, A.J. and Boime, I. (1989). Expression of biologically active human follitropin in Chinese hamster ovary cells. *J. Biol. Chem.*, **2640**, 4769–75

7. Hard, K., Mekking, A., Damm,. J.B., Kamerling, J.P., Boer, W., Wijnands, R.A. and Vliegenthart, J.F. (1990). Isolation and structure determination of the intact sialylated N-linked carbohydrate chains of recombinant human follitropin (hFSH) expressed in Chinese hamster ovary cells. *Eur. J. Biochem.*, **193**, 263–71

8. De Boer, W. and Mannaerts, B. (1990). Recombinant follicle stimulating hormone II. Biochemical and biological characteristics. In Crommelin, D.J.A. and Schellekens, H. (eds.) *From Clone to Clinic, Developments in Biotherapy*, pp. 253–9. (New York: Kluwer)

9. Mannaerts, B., De. Leeuw, R., Feelen, J., Van Ravenstein, A., Van Wezenbeek, P., Schuurs, A. and Kloosterboer, H. (1991). Comparative *in vitro* and *in vivo* studies on the biological properties of recombinant human follicle stimulating hormone. *Endocrinology*, **129**, 2623–30

10. Mannaerts, B., Shoham, Z., Schoot, D., Bouchard, P., Harlin, J., Fauser, B., Jacobs, H., Rombout, F. and Coelingh Bennink, H. (1993). Single-dose pharmacokinetics and pharmacodynamics of recombinant human follicle-stimulating hormone (Org 32489) in gonadotrophin-deficient volunteers. *Fertil. Steril.*, **59**, 108–14

11. Matikainen, T., De Leeuw, R., Mannaerts, B. and Huhtaniermi, I. (1993). Circulating bioactive and immunoreactive recombinant human follicle stimulating hormone (Org 32489) after administration to gonadotrophin-deficient subjects. *Fertil. Steril.*, **61**, 62–9

12. Schoot, B., Coelingh Bennink, H., Mannaerts, B., Lamberts, S., Bouchard, P. and Fauser, B.C. (1992). Human recombinant follicle-stimulating hormone induces growth of preovulatory follicles without concomitant increase in androgen and oestrogen biosynthesis in a woman with isolated gonadotrophin deficiency. *J. Clin. Endocrinol. Metab.*, **74**, 1471–3

13. Shoham, Z., Mannaerts, B., Insler, V. and Coelingh Bennink, H. (1993). Induction of follicular growth using recombinant human follicle-stimulating hormone in two volunteer women with hypogonadotropic hypogonadism. *Fertil. Steril.*, **59**, 738–42

14. Devroey, P., Mannaerts, B., Smitz, J., Coelingh Bennink, H., Van Steirteghem, A. (1993). First established pregnancy and birth after ovarian stimulation with recombinant human FSH (Org 32489). *Hum. Reprod.*, **8**, 863–5

15. Cochran, W. (1954). The combination of estimates from different experiments. *Biometrics*, **10**, 101–29

16. Whitehead, A. and Whitehead, J. (1991). A general parametric approach to the meta-analysis of randomised clinical trials. *Stat. Med.*, **10**, 1665–77

17. Out, H.J., Mannaerts, B.M.J.L. and Coelingh Bennink, H.J.T. (1994). A prospective, multicentre, randomized, assessor-blind study on the safety and efficacy of recombinant FSH (Org 32489, Puregon®) in IVF. *Hum. Reprod.*, **9** (Suppl. 3), 2

18. Rogers, M., Mitchell, R., Lambert, A., Peers, N., Roberts, W.R. and Robertson, C. (1992). Human chorionic gonadotrophin contributes to the bioactivity of Pergonal. *Clin. Endocrinol.*, **37**, 558–64

19. Council of Europe (1986). European Pharmacopoeia, 1986, 2nd edn., pp. 508.1–508.4

20. Steelman, S.L. and Pohley, F.M. (1953). Assay of the follicle stimulating hormone based on the augmentation with human chorionic gonadotropin. *Endocrinology*, **53**, 604–16

8

Ovarian hyperstimulation syndrome: prevention and management

N. Amso

INTRODUCTION

Ovarian hyperstimulation syndrome (OHSS) is an iatrogenic condition and remains the most serious and potentially lethal complication of ovulation induction. Its incidence varies with the different clinical conditions for which ovulation is induced, the gonadotrophin preparation administered, as well as the dosages and schedules. In contrast to OHSS during conventional ovulation induction, controlled ovarian hyperstimulation for assisted reproduction is a deliberate attempt to stimulate multiple follicular development, and rather than allowing for spontaneous follicular rupture, follicles are aspirated to retrieve the oocytes. During this process, intrafollicular haemorrhage may occur and any leakage into the peritoneal cavity may be mistaken for mild ascites. Additionally, reduction in granulosa cell content may have an immense effect on the quality of the ensuing luteal phase and on the prospect of OHSS.

RISK FACTORS

Young women, and those with polycystic ovaries, are known to be at greater risk. Similarly, OHSS correlates positively with conceptual cycles and is almost exclusively related to either exogenous or endogenous human chorionic gonadotrophin (hCG) stimulation. The incidence of the clinically severe form following *in vitro* fertilization (IVF) has been reported as being between 0.3 and 6%, the risk increasing with the total number of follicles in the preovulatory period, including immature and intermediate follicles. Furthermore, in the severe OHSS cases, 54.7% of the follicles have been reported to be < 9 mm in diameter[1]. The use of gonadotrophin releasing hormone agonist (GnRHa) in stimulation protocols has been reported to increase the incidence, although this is not universally accepted. Charbonnel and colleagues[2] detected OHSS in all patients who were treated with GnRHa and human menopausal gonadotrophin (hMG), 40% of which were moderate and 6% severe.

PATHOPHYSIOLOGY

The pathogenesis of OHSS is not yet fully understood. However, at the time of ovulation, several structural changes occur in the preovulatory follicle after the luteinizing hormone (LH) surge mediated by specific factors. These changes include an increase in ovarian blood flow, capillary fenestration and thecal oedema. It is also hypothesized that, in OHSS, there is marked peripheral arteriolar vasodilatation leading to underfilling of the arterial vascular compartment, arterial hypotension, and compensatory increase in heart rate and cardiac output[3]. An increase in capillary permeability of mesothelial surfaces also results in the massive ascites encountered in severe OHSS. Further evidence from animal studies suggests that isolation of the rabbit ovaries from the peritoneal cavity does not prevent ascites formation[4]. The resulting symptoms and physical signs are thus secondary to these major events. Corpus luteum activity also appears to be critical for the development of the syndrome. In its severe form there may be massive ovarian enlargement, ascites, pleural effusion, oliguria, electrolyte imbalance, haemoconcentration and hypercoagulability, and the condition is potentially fatal if not managed appropriately.

PRESENTATION AND CLASSIFICATION

OHSS may present 3–7 days after hCG injection (early presentation) or 12–17 days post-hCG (late presentation). The two modes of presentation rarely coexist. Stepwise logistic regression analysis[5] has shown that early

Table 1 Clinical classification of ovarian hyperstimulation syndrome

Grade	Findings
Mild	
1	Abdominal distension
2	Nausea, vomiting, diarrhoea, ovarian enlargement < 12 cm
Moderate	
3	Mild + ascites seen on scans
Severe	
4	Moderate + clinical evidence of ascites and hydrothorax, oliguria
5	Haemoconcentration, coagulation and electrolyte disorders, renal failure, respiratory distress, ovaries > 12 cm

OHSS is predicted by the number of oocytes retrieved and oestradiol concentration at the time of hCG administration. Late OHSS is predicted by the number of gestational sacs seen on ultrasound examination 4 weeks later only. Simply, early OHSS is an acute effect of the preovulatory dose of hCG, and late OHSS is induced by the rising serum concentration of hCG produced by early pregnancy.

A classification of OHSS based on clinical signs appears to be more appropriate than one defined purely by biochemical or ultrasound features[6]. It should also be remembered that a degree of hyperstimulation does occur when employing superovulation protocols for assisted reproduction, and mild or moderate forms are common. Ovarian size is an important parameter in determining severity when ovulation induction is the only treatment under consideration. However, in patients undergoing assisted reproduction treatment, thorough follicular aspiration results in ovaries that are not as enlarged as in the former case, and appropriate attention should be paid to the overall clinical picture as well as to a number of biochemical parameters. The presence of adult respiratory distress syndrome, tense ascites, severe haemoconcentration and profound leucocytosis are evidence of the severest life-threatening form. Table 1 summarizes the different grades of the disease and their corresponding clinical findings.

PREVENTION OF OHSS

The key to prevention is proper identification of the population at risk before treatment and close monitoring of hormone levels as well as multiple follicular response on ultrasound examination. Due to the difficulties in anticipating its occurrence, crude clinical and biological evaluation may be inadequate and more complex techniques such as multiple discriminant analysis may have to be employed to improve the prediction rate[7]. When a high-risk situation is recognized, withholding the ovulatory dose of hCG and cancellation of the treatment cycle will almost certainly prevent OHSS. The couple should be advised to avoid intercourse, as spontaneous ovulation may occur up to 11 days after discontinuing gonadotrophin treatment, resulting in conception and development of severe OHSS[8].

Alternative strategies usually succeed at ameliorating the severity of this complication, rather than its total prevention, and include eight distinct approaches. First, there may be reduction of the ovulatory hCG dose and avoidance of its use in the luteal phase. Second, triggering ovulation with GnRHa (intranasal or subcutaneous administration), instead of hCG, has been reported to have several advantages[9–11]. It simulates the natural LH and follicle stimulating hormone (FSH) surges; it does not affect the number of oocytes retrieved, fertilization or pregnancy rates, and furthermore, as the GnRHa has a short half-life, it does not exert any adverse effect on the luteal phase. However, moderate hyperstimulation may still occur if the patient conceives[12]. Such a protocol would be inapplicable for GnRHa superovulation protocols, and women with pituitary hypogonadotrophic amenorrhoea may show a weak response or none at all[12]. Future use of GnRH-antagonists may facilitate the widespread use of this approach.

A third strategy is that of alteration of ovarian response by reduction of the gonadotrophin dose in subsequent treatment cycles, which has been attempted with varying degrees of success. Pulsatile GnRH treatment or low-dose FSH stimulation regimens[13] have been reported to reduce the incidence of OHSS markedly. Forman and colleagues[14], in treatment cycles using GnRHa, continued with the analogue until full down-regulation and then restarted gonadotrophin injections at a lower dose without observing any cases of hyperstimulation. A review of the outcome of repeat treatment cycles in women whose previous cycles had been abandoned[15] showed cancellation in three of the 17 repeat cycles for fear of further hyperstimulation, and six of 11 oocyte collection cycles were associated with an exaggerated response, retrieving more than 11 oocytes in each case. A further three cycles failed to respond on the reduced dose completely.

A fourth approach, that of delaying the administration of hCG (controlled drift period or prolonged coasting) results in a rapid decline of oestradiol levels, but an increase in the size of the lead follicle and number of follicles > 14 mm in diameter. Clinical pregnancy rates between 25 and 35% have been reported[16,17]. However, in one study the multiple pregnancy rate was unacceptably high (50%) and severe OHSS occurred in 2.5% of all cases![17]

A fifth strategy involves conversion of a superovulation cycle with or without intrauterine insemination to *in vitro* fertilization and embryo transfer. This approach does not prevent the occurrence of OHSS following embryo transfer[18], but can help control against high-order multiple pregnancy.

A sixth approach is the elimination of the endogenous pregnancy-derived hCG by aspiration of all follicles, fertilization of oocytes and cryopreservation of all embryos. Transfer of frozen–thawed embryos in subsequent cycles has achieved very satisfactory pregnancy and implantation rates. In a previous publication by the present author and colleagues[19], it was demonstrated that the fertilization rate was not affected, luteal phase progress was not prolonged and the severity of the symptoms was moderate in most patients. Results from a larger number of patients confirmed earlier experience and showed that the quality of the embryos was not adversely affected, as manifested by the occurrence of pregnancies[20]. The improvement in the clinical symptoms corresponded with the decline in oestrogen and progesterone levels in the luteal phase. Wada and colleagues[21] reported similar results and, furthermore, achieved equal pregnancy rates following frozen–thawed embryo transfers in natural or hormone replacement therapy (HRT) cycles. Embryo replacement in natural cycles does not require any medication and is preferred for poorly compliant patients. Whilst HRT cycles are more expensive, they have a fixed schedule, requiring few hospital visits, and are more suited for women with irregular cycles. The group also reported that continuation of GnRHa in the luteal phase did not add extra benefit to the treatment cycle and was unnecessary[22]. In summary, elective cryopreservation of embryos in the at-risk group (clinical findings: oestradiol > 3500 pg/ml and ultrasound features) reduces the severity, but not the occurrence, of OHSS and has no adverse effect on the prospects of pregnancy at a later time.

A seventh alternative is the use of intravenous albumin infusion at the time of oocyte recovery, which has been recently reported to prevent the development of severe OHSS[23,24]. In their randomized placebo-controlled study, Shoham and colleagues[24] reported that no patient who had received human albumin solution developed severe OHSS, and hypothesized that albumin prevents this complication by binding an hCG-mediated factor secreted by the corpus luteum and which impedes capillary integrity. In addition, albumin is a highly effective plasma expander and thus reverses the hypovolaemia and haemoconcentration seen in OHSS.

A final, eighth strategy involves use of steroids in high-risk patients, which has been recently evaluated in a randomized study but was found to be ineffective in reducing the rate of OHSS after superovulation for IVF[25].

TREATMENT OF OHSS

Treatment of OHSS depends on its severity, the stage at which the diagnosis is made, and whether the patient is pregnant or not. In women with mild/moderate OHSS (haematocrit $\leq 44\%$), bed rest, increased fluid intake and close monitoring of the biochemical profile should be followed. This may be carried out without the need for admission to hospital. Patients with severe OHSS (haematocrit $\geq 45\%$; massive ascites) should be hospitalized and if critically ill should be cared for in intensive care units. Meticulous fluid and electrolyte balance should be maintained, using both crystalloids and colloids, until haemoconcentration abates. Monitoring of the progress of the disease should include close observation of haematocrit, urea and electrolytes, liver function tests, coagulation profile, and urine output[26].

Other methods have been proposed, including the use of antihistamines and indomethacin. Paracentesis, for symptomatic relief, failing renal function and reinfusion of ascitic fluid, with or without ultrafiltration, has also been reported[27,28]. Dramatic improvement in clinical symptoms may occur following paracentesis with almost instantaneous diuresis, decrease in haematocrit, improved creatinine clearance, and prevention of respiratory distress. Paracentesis (transabdominally or through the vaginal route) should not be performed without direct ultrasound guidance, if the patient is haemodynamically unstable, or if there is suspected haemoperitoneum. In an extreme situation, therapeutic interruption of an early pregnancy may be the only lifesaving action, when other measures have failed.

CONCLUSIONS

In summary, ovarian hyperstimulation syndrome may not be totally avoidable in assisted reproduction treatment, and in view of the continuing uncertainty surrounding its pathophysiology, as well as the seriousness of this complication, clinicians must ensure due attention to the risk factors and strict monitoring of ovulation induction techniques. A clear plan for the management of this complication should be formulated, subject to the available resources, in each assisted reproduction institution and couples must be informed of this potentially fatal complication before the initiation of treatment.

REFERENCES

1. Blankstein, J., Shalev, J., Saadon, T., Kukia, E.E., Rabinovici, J., Pariente, C., Lunenfeld, B., Serr, D.M. and Mashiach, S. (1987). Ovarian hyperstimulation syndrome: prediction by number and size of preovulatory ovarian follicles. *Fertil. Steril.*, **47**, 597–602
2. Charbonnel, B., Krempf, M., Blanchard, P., Dano, F. and Delage, C. (1987). Induction of ovulation in polycystic ovary syndrome with a combination of a luteinizing hormone-releasing hormone analog and exogenous gonadotropins. *Fertil. Steril.*, **47**, 920–9
3. Balasch, J., Arroyo, V., Carmona, F., Llach, J., Jimenez, W., Pare, J.C. and Vanrell, J.A. (1991). Severe ovarian hyperstimulation syndrome: role of peripheral vasodilation. *Fertil. Steril.*, **56**, 1077–83
4. Yarali, H., Fleige-Zahradka, B.G., Yuen, B.H. and McComb, P.F. (1993). The ascites in the ovarian hyperstimulation syndrome does not originate from the ovary. *Fertil. Steril.*, **59**, 657–61
5. Dahl Lyons, C., Wheeler, C.A., Frishman, G.N., Hackett, R.J., Seifer,

D.B. and Haning, R.V. (1994). Early and late presentation of the ovarian hyperstimulation syndrome: two distinct entities with different risk factors. *Hum. Reprod.*, **9**, 792–9

6. Golan, A., Ron-El, R., Soffer, Y., Weinraub, Z. and Caspi, E. (1989). Ovarian hyperstimulation syndrome: An update review. *Obstet. Gynecol. Surv.*, **6**, 430–40

7. Delvigne, A., Dubois, M., Battheu, B., Bassil, S., Meuleman, C., De Sutter, P., Rodesch, C., Janssens, P., Remacle, P., Gordts, S., Puttemans, P., Joostens, M., van Roosendaal, E. and Leroy, F. (1993). The ovarian hyperstimulation syndrome in *in-vitro* fertilization: a Belgian multicentric study. II. Multiple discriminant analysis for risk prediction. *Hum. Reprod.*, **8**, 1361–6

8. Lipitz, S., Ben-Rafael, Z., Bider, D., Shalev, J. and Mashiach, S. (1991). Quintuplet pregnancy and third degree ovarian hyperstimulation despite withholding human chorionic gonadotrophin. *Hum. Reprod.*, **6**, 1478–9

9. Imoedemhe, D.A., Chan, R.C., Sigue, A.B., Pacpaco, E.L. and Olazo, A.B. (1991). A new approach to the management of patients at risk of ovarian hyperstimulation in an *in-vitro* fertilization programme. *Hum. Reprod.*, **6**, 1088–91

10. Gonen, Y., Balakier, H., Powell, W. and Casper, F.R.F. (1990). Use of gonadotropin-releasing hormone agonist to trigger follicular maturation for *in vitro* fertilization. *J. Clin. Endocrinol. Metab.*, **71**, 918–22

11. Shalev, E., Geslevich, Y. and Ben-Ami, M. (1994). Induction of pre-ovulatory luteinizing hormone surge by gonadotrophin-releasing hormone agonist for women at risk for developing the ovarian hyperstimulation syndrome. *Hum. Reprod.*, **9**, 417–19

12. van der Meer, S., Gerris, J., Joostens, M. and Tas, B. (1993). Triggering of ovulation using a gonadotrophin-releasing hormone agonist does not prevent ovarian hyperstimulation syndrome. *Hum. Reprod.*, **8**, 1628–31

13. Dale, P.O., Tanbo, T., Haug, E. and Åbyholm, T. (1992). Polycystic ovary syndrome: low-dose follicle stimulating hormone administration is a safe stimulation regimen even in previous hyper-responsive patients. *Hum. Reprod.*, **7**, 1085–9

14. Forman, R.G., Frydman, R., Egan, D., Ross, C. and Barlow, D. (1990). Severe ovarian hyperstimulation syndrome using agonists of gonadotropin-releasing hormone for *in vitro* fertilization: a European series and a proposal for prevention. *Fertil. Steril.*, **53**, 502–9

15. Amso, N.N., Shaw, R.W., Ahuja, K.K. and Morris, N. (1991). Prevention of ovarian hyperstimulation syndrome (letter). *Fertil. Steril.*, **55**, 220–1

16. Sher, G., Salem, R., Feinman, M., Dodge, S., Zouves, C. and Knutzen, V. (1993). Eliminating the risk of life-endangering complications following

overstimulation with menotropin fertility agents: a report on women undergoing *in vitro* fertilization and embryo transfer. *Obstet. Gynecol.*, **81**, 1009–11

17. Urman, B., Pride, S.M. and Yuen, B.H. (1992). Management of overstimulated gonadotrophin cycles with a controlled drift period. *Hum. Reprod.*, **7**, 213–17

18. Nisker, J., Tummon, I., Daniel, S., Kaplan, B. and Yuzpe, A. (1994). Conversion of cycles involving hyperstimulation with intrauterine insemination to *in-vitro* fertilization. *Hum. Reprod.*, **9**, 406–8

19. Amso, N.N., Ahuja, K., Morris, N. and Shaw, R.W. (1990). The management of ovarian hyperstimulation involving gonadotropin releasing hormone analogue with elective cryopreservation of all embryos. *Fertil. Steril.*, **53**, 1087–90

20. Amso, N. and Shaw, R.W. (1991). Polycystic ovaries and problems in assisted reproduction programmes. In Shaw, R.W. (ed.) *Polycystic Ovaries: a Disorder or a Symptom?*, pp. 203–216. (Carnforth, UK: Parthenon Publishing)

21. Wada, I., Matson, P.L., Troup, S.A., Hughes, S., Buck, P. and Lieberman, B.A. (1992). Outcome of treatment subsequent to the elective cryopreservation of all embryos from women at risk of the ovarian hyperstimulation syndrome. *Hum. Reprod.*, **7**, 962–6

22. Wada, I., Matson, P.L., Horne, G., Buck, P. and Lieberman, B.A. (1992). Is continuation of a gonadotrophin-releasing hormone agonist (GnRHa) necessary for women at risk of developing the ovarian hyperstimulation syndrome?. *Hum. Reprod.*, **7**, 1090–3

23. Asch, R.H., Ivery, G., Goldsman, M., Frederick, J.L., Stone, S.C. and Balmaceda, J.P. (1993). The use of intravenous albumin in patients at high risk for severe ovarian hyperstimulation syndrome. *Hum. Reprod.*, **8**, 1015–20

24. Shoham, Z., Weissman, A., Barash, A., Borenstein, R., Schachter, M. and Insler, V. (1994). Intravenous albumin for the prevention of severe ovarian hyperstimulation syndrome in an *in vitro* fertilization programme: a prospective, randomized, placebo-controlled study. *Fertil. Steril.*, **62**, 137–42

25. Tan, S.L., Balen, A., el Hussein, E., Campbell, S. and Jacobs, H.S. (1992). The administration of glucocorticoids for the prevention of ovarian hyperstimulation syndrome in *in vitro* fertilization: a prospective randomized study. *Fertil. Steril.*, **58**, 378–83

26. Navot, D., Bergh, P.A. and Laufer, N. (1992). Ovarian hyperstimulation syndrome in novel reproductive technologies: prevention and treatment. *Fertil. Steril.*, **58**, 249–61

27. Aboulghar, M.A., Mansour, R.T., Serour, G.I., Riad, R. and Ramzi, A.M. (1992). Autotransfusion of the ascitic fluid in the treatment of severe ovarian hyperstimulation syndrome. *Fertil. Steril.*, **58**, 1056–9

28. Fukaya, T., Chida, S., Terada, Y., Funayama, Y. and Yajima, A. (1994). Treatment of severe ovarian hyperstimulation syndrome by ultrafiltration and reinfusion of ascitic fluid. *Fertil. Steril.*, **61**, 561–4

9

Micromanipulation techniques: male infertility resolved?

S. Green, S.B. Fishel, J.A. Hall, S. Fleming, A.J. Hunter, K. Dowell and S. Thornton

INTRODUCTION

Defining male infertility is complex because it can be related to conception *in vivo* or *in vitro*. Male infertility can be defined according to abnormal semen characteristics which may be associated with chromosomal, genetic, structural or endocrine dysfunction or which are completely unrelated to any known cause. Sub-microscopic sperm dysfunction (e.g. receptors, acrosomal contents, flagella activity, etc.) is not always associated with defects in contemporary measurements of seminal parameters such as density, motility, morphology and seminal biochemistry. A number of approaches, both diagnostic and technical, have been developed over the years to overcome male factor infertility.

Diagnostic sperm function tests, such as the acrosome reaction, ionophore challenge (ARIC) test, zona free hamster penetration test, measurement of oxygen free radicals, computer-assisted sperm analysis, pentoxifylline challenge tests, and so on, utilize biochemical and functional markers for fertility. To obtain a clear assessment of these test results one needs to know if a particular finding is permanent and reproducible. If the data are to be useful to the clinician and practising embryologist, they should offer a direction as to the appropriate type of assisted conception approach. At the present time the information from such diagnostic andrology is of limited value to the clinician and clinical embryologist. Some examples of sperm function tests are shown in Table 1.

Table 1 Sperm function tests

Test	Comment
Acrosome reaction	Using fluorescent staining (chlortetracycline – CTC fluorescein isothiocyanate Con A); resting state is compared to activated conditions
Binding to zona pellucida	Hemizona assay: two halves of same zona are used to measure binding of fertile donor sperm compared with test sperm (or a competitive test to whole zona)
Acrosomal enzyme (acrosin) assay	Area of gelatin digestion by capacitated sperm – a proteolytic assay Measurement of acrosin by ELISA
Sperm–oocyte fusion	Hamster egg penetration assay
Sperm capacitation	Computerized measurement of hyperactivation
Sperm morphology	Visualization of stained sperm Computerized evaluation
Chromosome analysis	Using decondensed sperm heads in hamster-egg assay (on chemically decondensed heads); *in situ* hybridization
Sperm viability	Dye exclusion tests
Sperm membrane stability	Hypo-osmotic swelling test
Energy availability	Assessment of sperm ATP using bioluminescence
Excess lipid peroxidase	Measurement of reactive oxygen species
Immunological	Antisperm antibody assessment

The approaches used to treat male factor infertility are shown in Table 2; the most appropriate single or combined approach is often reached from the following information:

(1) Diagnostic andrology.

(2) Patient fertility history.

(3) Semen characteristics; strict morphology; total motile count; motility.

(4) Available oocyte numbers.

(5) Experience with similar problems in other patients.

(6) Discussion with couple.

GAMETE INTRAFALLOPIAN TRANSFER (GIFT)

This describes the transfer of an admixture of gametes to the Fallopian tube, after recovery of the oocytes either by laparoscopy or ultrasound-guided transvaginal follicular aspiration. This approach has proved successful for many thousands of patients with unexplained infertility. GIFT has been used successfully as a treatment for moderate cases of oligozoospermia of $> 5 \times 10^6 \, \mathrm{ml^{-1}}$ and teratozoospermia, $\leq 14\%$ normal forms[1,2].

CONVENTIONAL *IN VITRO* FERTILIZATION (IVF)

Many units still prefer conventional IVF (insemination with 50 000 to 100 000 motile sperm), to GIFT for male factor cases, In part, this is because transvaginal oocyte recovery, and not laparoscopy, is used, but mainly because much more information is available from IVF, such as oocyte morphology, degree of oocyte maturity, fertilization potential, embryo morphology, etc.

At NURTURE (Nottingham University Research and Treatment Unit in Reproduction), for example, the authors have treated by IVF more than 100 patients who had previously failed to achieve pregnancy after one or more attempts at GIFT. In each case an *in vitro* fertilization problem was apparent due to gamete dysfunction.

Table 2 Assisted reproduction techniques and procedures available for male infertility. GIFT, gamete intrafallopian transfer; HIC, high insemination concentration; ICSI, intracytoplasmic sperm injection; IVF, *in vitro* fertilization; μIVF, micro-drop *in vitro* fertilization; SUZI, subzonal insemination

Procedure	Comment
Drugs	Gonadotrophins
	Anti-oestrogens
	Androgens
	Vitamin E
	Motility enhancement
	Methylxanthines
	Corticosteroids
Surgery	Varicocoele
	Vasectomy reversal / other anastomotic surgery
	Epididymal aspiration
	Testicular biopsy
Cryopreservation of sperm	Moderate oligo / normal asthenozoospermia
	Epididymal sperm (congenital absence of vas)
GIFT	Mild–moderate oligo / astheno / teratozoospermia
IVF conventional	Mild–moderate oligo / astheno / teratozoospermia
IVF modified	
(a) HIC	Severe teratozoospermia
	Moderate teratozoospermia if previous failed IVF
(b) μIVF	Very severe oligo- and / or asthenozoospermia
(c) μIVF / HIC combination	Very severe oligo- and / or astheno / teratozoospermia

(*continued*)

Table 2 *continued*

Procedure	Comment
Micro–assisted fertilization	
(a) SUZI	Failed IVF / modified IVF (especially with failed binding to zona pellucida) with or without severe seminal defects
(b) ICSI	As for SUZI plus spermatogenic arrest, Kartagener / immotile cilia syndrome, total immotile sperm, testicular sperm, extreme (100%) teratozoospermia, globozoospermia

The first observation that IVF could procure conception in *in vitro* cases of severe oligozoospermia was made in 1991[3]. Further studies have proved the value of this approach in men with varying types of single or multiple seminal defects[4–6]. However, the degree of severity of oligozoospermia, asthenozoospermia and teratozoospermia is not clear from these papers, and workers have noted a reduction in the incidence of fertilization when using IVF with these types of sperm defects. One of the most predictive factors for IVF is sperm morphology, particularly using the strict criteria[7]. This analysis indicates a fertilization prognosis of < 10%, where there is a normal morphology figure of < 5%, and a 64% fertilization prognosis where normal morphology lies between 5 and 14%[7]. However, the success of conventional IVF in treating the severe male forms of infertility is limited and, consequently, further mechanical and technical procedures have been devised.

MODIFICATIONS OF IVF

High insemination concentration IVF (HIC)

In some patients who have an acceptable sperm count and motility, with or without varying degrees of teratozoospermia, but who have previously failed to achieve fertilization, it is possible to procure fertilization by modifying the insemination concentration.

We have achieved fertilization and successful embryo cleavage leading to clinical pregnancy and delivery by performing HIC insemination with > 200 000 motile sperm per ml, but usually not exceeding $1 \times 10^6\,\text{ml}^{-1}$, depending on strict morphology and history. This is a useful technique in patients referred for micro-assisted fertilization with normal semen parameters, but with a history of repeated failure at conventional IVF. More recently, we have observed a certain group of patients where the percentage fertilization is improved using HIC[8]. Table 3 shows the use of HIC in ten cases of asthenozoospermia with previous failure of IVF.

Microdrop IVF (μIVF)

In cases of severe oligozoospermia and/or asthenozoospermia it is sometimes possible to procure fertilization by careful concentration of the available motile sperm in a microdrop (5 μl). The oocytes are removed from the cumulus oophorus using hyaluronidase and placed in a microdrop of sperm suspension. The effect is to increase substantially the gamete ratio; to effect this, however, the sperm may need to be concentrated into a volume too small to accept a single cumulus oophorous.

The advantages of using modified IVF procedures in the procurement of fertilization in male infertility are technical, financial, and of prognostic value. If IVF embryos are produced and embryo morphology is acceptable, in general these embryos are transferred in preference, as implantation rates are higher and uncertainties still remain about the long-term safety of micro-injected embryos. Alternatively, patients have the option to have MAF embryos transferred and IVF embryos cryopreserved, since IVF embryo thawing rates are often higher than those of MAF-derived embryos[9]. The decision to use these procedures is undertaken very carefully and in consultation with the couple. In cases of teratozoospermia a combination of IVF and HIC may be used on a cohort of oocytes. Often, a combined approach of micro-assisted fertilization (MAF) and modified IVF is useful at the first attempt, provided there is a large enough cohort of oocytes. Following a failure of fertilization, re-insemination with a known fertile donor, as a test only, can be a useful indicator of gamete dysfunction. Knowledge of the *in vitro* fertilization potential may affect future management of the problem and significantly alter the financial commitment faced by the couple.

Table 3 The use of high insemination concentration (HIC) in ten cases of asthenozoospermia with previous failure of *in vitro* fertilization. ICSI, intracytoplasmic sperm injection; SUZI, subzonal insemination

Patient No.	Total motile count ($\times 10^6$)	% Normal morphology	No. oocytes fertilized / No. inseminated		No. HIC embryos transferred	Outcome
			SUZI / ICSI★	HIC		
1	64	7	3/7	5/5	3	Delivery × 1
2	115	1	1/4	3/4	3	Delivery × 2
3	32	5	2/7	2/3	2 + 1 ICSI	Miscarriage 10 weeks: 2 sacs
4	25	9	2/18	6/10	3	Delivery × 1
5	17	2	0/4	2/4	2	Delivery × 1
6	61	6	0/6	1/3	1	Miscarriage 8 weeks
7	42	5	3/8	4/8	2 + 1 SUZI	Miscarriage 12 weeks: 2 sacs
8	29	4	3/4	1/3	1 + 2 SUZI	Ongoing: 3 sacs
9	31	4	3/6	3/5	2 + 1 SUZI	Ongoing: 2 sacs
10	18	3	4/4	3/4	3	Ongoing: 1 sac

★sibling oocytes

MICRO-ASSISTED FERTILIZATION APPROACHES TO MALE INFERTILITY

The clinical application of micro-insemination techniques was first reported in 1985[10]; the use of subzonal insemination (SUZI) in 1987[11], and intracytoplasmic sperm injection (ICSI) in 1988[12]. Other zona-breaching studies were reported in 1988[13]. In the same year, implantation of human embryos after partial zona dissection (PZD) was reported for the first time[14]. In 1988, the first pregnancy after SUZI was also reported[15], followed in 1990 by the first published birth of a set of twins and a singleton after SUZI[16]. In 1992 a high incidence of fertilization and pregnancy after ICSI was reported[17,18]. This procedure has been heralded as the main revolution in the treatment of male factor infertility. At the time of writing, NURTURE is currently reporting the birth of the first baby conceived after SUZI where oocyte fertilization resulted from a technique termed 'computer image sperm selection' (CISS)[19].

ZONA BREACHING

Zona puncture (ZP) and partial zona dissection (PZD)

The zona pellucida is the acellular physical barrier of the oocyte presented to the sperm, and there have been numerous approaches to breaching this barrier. The first approach was to use a chemical or an enzyme, such as chymotrypsin, to digest a path through the zona. Although fertilization can be achieved by these means, results were poor and this approach has now ceased as a viable option in humans. Manual methods of breaching the zona have been partial zona dissection (PZD) and zona puncture (ZP) using microneedles which create pathways for the sperm to swim through and approach the egg directly. In zona puncture the microneedle is inserted to create a large hole, often through the opposing zona, and simply retracted. In PZD the oocyte is removed from the holding pipette after puncture, and while the microneedle still pierces the opposite sides of the zona it is rubbed against the holding needle until it tears. After this manipulation the oocytes are inseminated in the same manner as with IVF. There is considerable debate about the value of these methods. After the first pregnancy was reported using zona breaching in 1988[14], proponents of the PZD method reported some remarkable increases in the incidence of fertilization and pregnancy.

Some units were not successful with these approaches and some reports showed that by simply modifying IVF, such as the HIC approach, successful conception could be achieved. Fishel and colleagues[20] published results showing that PZD proved successful in patients who had had only one failure at IVF, but was unsuccessful if there were multiple failures at IVF. Tucker and co-workers[21], however, abandoned the use of PZD as being too inconsistent and many centres have now done the same.

Subzonal insemination (SUZI)

The zona-breaching procedures, such as PZD, depend on the inherent motility of spermatozoa. They have been moderately successful in treating various degrees of oligozoospermia, asthenozoospermia, teratozoospermia, unexplained failure of fertilization, failure of binding to the zona and the presence of antisperm antibodies. Results, however, have been inconsistent. Subzonal insemination of sperm provided a means of breaching the zona which provided better and more consistent results and has been used to treat the anomalies listed above and, moreover, very severe asthenozoospermia and very severe oligozoospermia. As with the zona puncture and PZD techniques, SUZI requires the oocyte to be stripped of the corona radiata. A number of sperm are then inserted into the perivitelline space. Many studies have been published which have utilized zona breaching – mainly PZD and SUZI procedures. In contrast to the findings of PZD, the fertilization rate using SUZI in couples with a history of multiple failures of IVF was higher[22,23]. In 1993, in a comparison between the use of SUZI and PZD in the same patient, it was shown that SUZI resulted in a significantly higher fertilization rate[23]. The benefit of PZD decreased for patients with lower than 600 000 sperm in the ejaculate, and PZD was of no benefit to patients who required epididymal aspiration[23].

Several workers have found that multiple sperm can be injected into the perivitelline space without an extraordinary increase in polyspermy. This has been suggested to correlate with the incidence of abnormal forms in the ejaculate[24]. There have been striking differences reported between groups in the incidence of polyspermy as the number of sperm injected into the perivitelline space increases[22,25–28]. There is probably a degree of block to polyspermy at the level of the vitelline membrane and there may be a correlation with the numbers of abnormal forms. This observation, however, may also be due to the effect of manually selecting spermatozoa for the SUZI method, some or all of which may not have the potential to fertilize. Table 4 illustrates a comparison of the techniques of SUZI and PZD vs. µIVF in ten cases of severe oligozoospermia and/or asthenozoospermia with previous failure of IVF.

Computer image sperm selection (CISS)

Within our own unit, as part of an ongoing research programme, we have been examining the potential for standardizing the SUZI method by selecting sperm capable of acrosome reacting and fusing. To do this we have been using real-time computer-assisted sperm analysis (CASA) analysis of individual sperm in a micro-injection environment: a technique we have called 'computer image sperm selection' (CISS). Hyperactivation is regarded as a marker for successful capacitation and a precursor to the acrosome reaction. The 'Hobson Sperm Tracker' (Hobson Tracking Systems Ltd., Sheffield, UK) observes and visibly highlights sperm which satisfy these criteria. In a pilot study of patients treated by the SUZI technique with and without CISS, the results showed a significant increase in the fertilization rate overall with a tenfold increase in polyspermy when CISS was used – with up to one-third less sperm than for conventional SUZI[19]. The overall fertilization rate, including that of monospermy, doubled.

Variations in pregnancy rates with the conventional approach to SUZI have been published. In cases of repeated failure of conventional or modified IVF, delivery rates have been approximately 10–15%. To improve on this, the overall incidence of fertilization per oocyte (currently 15–25%) must be increased.

The use of very low numbers of selected sperm, or even a single sperm, using the CISS method, delivered either into the perivitelline space or an invagination in the vitelline membrane, may result in a more controlled fertilization prognosis from the SUZI technique. This more physiological approach might improve the efficiency of conception and implantation rates.

Table 4 The use of subzonal insemination (SUZI) and partial zona dissection (PZD) vs. micro-drop *in vitro* fertilization (µIVF) in ten cases of severe oligo- and / or asthenozoospermia with previous failure of IVF

Patient No.	Total motile count ($\times 10^6$)	No. oocytes fertilized / No. inseminated		No. µIVF embryos transferred	Outcome
		SUZI / PZD★	µIVF		
1	4	5 / 8	4 / 4	3	Delivery × 1
2	9	1 / 13	3 / 4	3	Delivery × 1
3	2	3 / 6	2 / 3	2 + 1 PZD	Delivery × 2
4	3	0 / 4	2 / 4	2	Delivery × 1
5	1	0 / 3	1 / 3	1	Miscarriage 9 weeks
6	7	2 / 8	3 / 3	3	Delivery × 1
7	2	1 / 10	2 / 4	2 + 1 PZD	Delivery × 1 Miscarriage 7 weeks × 1
8	1	3 / 9	3 / 5	3	Ongoing × 2
9	4	4 / 6	3 / 6	3	Ongoing × 1
10	4	2 / 7	4 / 6	3	Ongoing × 2

★ sibling oocytes

INTRACYTOPLASMIC SPERM INJECTION (ICSI)

Although there have been many animal experiments with ICSI, until 1992 it was considered too invasive to be used for human fertility treatment. The 1992 report by Palermo and colleagues[17], comparing SUZI and ICSI in couples with severely impaired sperm characteristics, proved to be the turning point in clinical micro-injection technology. In this report 66% of 47 oocytes were fertilized and four pregnancies resulted from eight treatment cycles; two healthy boys were delivered from singleton pregnancies and a boy and a girl from a twin pregnancy[17]. Largely based on this publication, and on those of Van Steirteghem and co-workers[29,30], this technique has gained worldwide acceptance as probably the ultimate micro-assisted fertilization approach for all cases requiring micro-injection technology. Tables 5 and 6 show the results using ICSI.

Data from a number of groups who now have experience with ICSI demonstrate that high fertilization and pregnancy rates can be achieved. However, the success of ICSI is related more to good technique than to other micro-assisted fertilization approaches. Some of the technical difficulties have been illustrated[34]. Three locations for the sperm after ICSI have been demonstrated: first, within the perivitelline space (indicating no piercing of the inner membrane); second, within oolemma-bound vacuoles in the peripheral ooplasm (created by invagination and pocketing of the oolemma); and third, lying free in the ooplasm. Recent ICSI data from Fishel and colleagues[35] demonstrated fertilization in patients with 100% immotile sperm, globozoospermia, spermatogenic arrest and testicular sperm, and it is this procedure that has been the first to achieve a pregnancy with sperm recovered directly from the testis[23]. Although ICSI treatment of globozoospermia has resulted in fertilization, these sperm have a centrally located chromatin defect in the head and, at the time of writing, no viable pregnancies have been reported. Fertilization rates in excess of 50% and pregnancy rates between 15 and 35% have been achieved with the ICSI method.

Tucker and co-workers[21] reported that their ICSI approach yielded results comparable only to conventional SUZI; however, our data are in accordance with others showing significantly higher sucess rates, fertilization and pregnancy with ICSI[29,30]. Our current research centres on ICSI with the immature spermatozoon or the spermatid, an approach which is feasible, as pronuclei have been formed in a cell-free lysate

Table 5 Current published data from studies using intracytoplasmic sperm injection. SUZI, subzonal insemination

Group	Incidence of monospermic fertilization (n = oocytes)	Incidence of ongoing pregnancies (n = embryo transfers)	Comments
Van Steirteghem et al.[30]	47% (n = 3944)	28% (n = 350)	Previous failed fertilization or with < 5% of oocytes fertilized, and male factor
Fishel et al.[31]	28% (n = 251)	20% (n = 20)	Failed SUZI on two previous occasions, extreme male factor, including globozoospermia
Gianaroli et al.[32]	42% (n = 115)	15% (n = 13)	'Extremely severe male factor' (no details)
Hamberger et al.[33]	53% (n = 782)	32% (n = 63)	No details on patient selection

Table 6 Fifty-nine cases of extreme male factor infertility treated by intracytoplasmic sperm injection. ET, embryo transfer

	No. of patients with fertilization / total no. of patients	No. of oocytes fertilized / no. of oocytes	Outcome
Spermatogenic arrest	14 / 17 (82%)	35 / 119 (29%)	14 patients with ET: five ongoing pregnancies
Testicular sperm	4 / 4 (100%)	12 / 38 (32%)	Four patients with ET: one ongoing pregnancy
Globozoospermia	5 / 13 (38%)	16 / 90 (18%)	Five patients with ET: no pregnancy
100% immotile sperm	9 / 16 (56%)	29 / 175 (17%)	Nine patients with ET: two ongoing pregnancies
Kartagener syndrome	7 / 9 (78%)	29 / 63 (46%)	Six patients with ET: no pregnancy

system[36], and mice have been born after the use of spermatids for conception[37].

LASER BEAM TECHNOLOGY

Laser beam technology was first introduced into micromanipulation techniques in 1989[38]. Gamete micromanipulation requires precise micro-tools and, consequently, the use of laser light for cutting the zona pellucida, or trapping and moving spermatozoa is an attractive alternative. This type of approach has been discussed in detail elsewhere[39]. However, the current high cost of these procedures will delay the necessary detailed evaluation.

TOTAL PREGNANCIES WORLDWIDE RESULTING FROM MICROMANIPULATION TECHNIQUES

The most comprehensive survey to date is based on 27 units utilizing micro-assisted fertilization[40]. Of the 971 pregnancies established (353 ICSI) 426 have been delivered with six (1.4%) major malformations reported. Of the 353 ICSI pregnancies, 91 babies have been delivered to date. There has been one case of hydro-anencephalus in twins, each one with cleft palate, and one delivery with a cleft lip and palate with duplication of urinary collecting system. Of the 228 babies from 453 SUZI pregnancies reported to date, one trisomy 16 which miscarried represents the only data available. Of the 137 pregnancies resulting from the use of PZD, there have been 93 babies to date, one of which had anencephaly. Further detailed studies of all births are advisable until many more infants have resulted from micro-assisted fertilization techniques.

SUMMARY

Conventional and modified IVF (high insemination concentration and microdrop IVF) are being used successfully to procure conception *in vitro* and the birth of normal children to couples with mild to moderately severe conditions of male factor infertility. Micromanipulation procedures are becoming more successful, notwithstanding the almost universally accepted decline in the use of partial zona dissection. Subzonal insemination and intracytoplasmic sperm injection are the preferred techniques, with the probability that subzonal insemination (perhaps incorporating computer image sperm selection) will be used in a few selected patients, particularly those with few or fragile oocytes (not all oocytes are expected to survive ICSI), or those holding ethical or religious objections to ICSI itself. Although concerns of safety still exist, these have now been somewhat alleviated by current data, but vigilance still needs to be maintained.

Male infertility resolved?

The technical advances in the approach to the treatment of male factor infertility have been dramatic in recent years. The efficacy of these procedures will improve as our knowledge of sperm function increases and as our technical expertise increases. Perhaps urological surgery and all other approaches to date will be redundant in the face of micromanipulation and computer technology.

ACKNOWLEDGEMENTS

Our thanks, as always, to Rosie Metcalf and Christine Poyser for helping in the preparation of this manuscript.

REFERENCES

1. Matson, P.L., Blackledge, D.G. and Richardson, P.A. (1987). The role of gamete intra-fallopian transfer (GIFT) in the treatment of oligospermic infertility. *Fertil. Steril.*, **48**, 608–23
2. Cittadini, E., Guastella, G., Comparetto, G., Gattucio, F. and Chianchiano, N. (1988). IVF-ET and GIFT in andrology. *Hum. Reprod.*, **3**, 101–4
3. Kavella, M., Lipovac, V. and Marotti, T. (1991). Effect of pentoxifylline on superoxide and anion production by human sperm. *Int. J. Androl.*, **14**, 320–7
4. Cohen, J., Edwards, R.G., Fahealy, C.B. and Fishel, S.B. (1984). Treatment of male infertility by *in-vitro* fertilisation. Factors affecting fertilisation and pregnancy. *Acta Eur. Fertil.*, **15**, 455–65

5. Gibbons, W. (1987). *In-vitro* fertilisation as a therapy for male-factor infertility. *Urol. Clin. North Am.*, **14**, 563–7

6. Yates, C.A. and de Kretser, D.M. (1987). Male factor infertility *in vitro* fertilisation. *J. In Vitro Fertil. Embryo Transfer* **4**, 141–7

7. Kruger, T.F., Acosta, A.A. and Simmons, K.F. (1988). Predicted value of abnormal sperm morphology in IVF. *Fertil. Steril.*, **49**, 112–17

8. Fishel, S.B., Hall, J.A., Timson, J.A., Green, S., Fleming, S. and Thornton, S. (1994). High concentration IVF for 29 cases of very severe teratozoospermia. Presented at the *Society for the Study of Fertility*, July, Southampton

9. Van Steirteghem, A.C., Van der Elst, J., Van den Abbeel, E., Joris, H., Camus, M. and Devroey, P. (1994). Cryopreservation of supernumerary multicellular human embryos obtained after intracytoplasmic sperm injection. *Fertil. Steril.*, **62**, 775–80

10. Metka, M., Haromy, T., Huber, J. and Shurz, B. (1985). Artificial insemination using a micromanipulator. *Fertilitat.* **1**, 41–7

11. Laws-King, A., Trounson, A., Sathananthan, H. and Kola, I. (1987). Fertilisation of human oocytes by micro-injection of a single spermatozoon under the zona pellucida. *Fertil. Steril.*, **48**, 637–42

12. Lanzendorf, E., Maloney, M.K. and Veek, L.L. (1988). A preclinical evaluation of human spermatozoa into human oocytes. *Fertil. Steril.*, **49**, 835–42

13. Gordon, J.W., Grunfeld, J., Garrisi, G.J., Talansky, B.E., Richards, C. and Lowfer, N. (1988). Fertilisation of human oocytes by sperm from infertile males after zona pellucida drilling. *Fertil. Steril.*, **50**, 673–83

14. Cohen, J., Malta, M., Fehilly, C., Wright, G., Elsner, C., Kort, H. and Massey, J. (1988). Implantation of embryos after partial opening of oocyte zona pellucida to facilitate sperm penetration. *Lancet*, **2**, 162

15. Ng, S.-C., Bongso, T.A., Ratnam, S.S., Sathananthan, A.H., Chan, C.L.K., Wong, P.C., Hagglund, L., Anandakumar, C., Wong, Y.C. and Coh, V.H.H. (1988). Pregnancy after transfer of multiple sperm under the zona. *Lancet*, **2**, 790

16. Fishel, S.B., Antinori, S., Jackson, P., Johnson, J., Lisi, F., Chiariello, F. and Versaci, C. (1990). Twin birth after subzonal insemination. *Lancet*, **2**, 722

17. Palermo, G., Joris, H., Devroey, P. and Van Steirteghem, A.C. (1992). Pregnancies after intracytoplasmic injection of single spermatozoon into an oocyte. *Lancet*, **340**, 17–18

18. Palermo, G., Joris, H., Derde, M-P, Devroey, P. and Van Steirteghem, A.C. (1993). Sperm characteristics and outcome of human assisted fertilisation by sub-zonal insemination and intracytoplasmic sperm injection. *Fertil. Steril.*, **59**, 826–35

19. Green, S., Fishel, S.B., Hall, J.A., Hunter, A.J., Fleming, S., Hobson, G., Roe, H., Dowell, K., Thornton, S. and Klentzeris, L. (1995). Computer

Image Sperm Selection (CISS) as a novel approach to sub-zonal insemination. *Hum. Reprod.*, in press

20. Fishel, S., Dowell, K., Timson, J., Green, S., Hall, J. and Klentzeris, L. (1993). Micro-assisted fertilisation with human gametes. *Hum. Reprod.*, **8**, 1780–4

21. Tucker, M., Weiker, S. and Massey, J. (1993). Rational approach to assisted fertilisation. *Hum. Reprod.*, **8**, 1778–85

22. Sakkas, D., Lacham, O., Giarnoli, L. and Trounson, A. (1991). Preliminary results on the comparison of sperm micro-injection and partial zona dissection as a treatment of male factor infertility. Presented at the *7th Meeting of the ESHRE and 7th World Congress on IVF and Assisted Procreation*, Paris

23. Vanderzwalmen, P., Burtin, G., Nijs, M. and Schoysman, R. (1993). Value of partial zona dissection for couples suffering from male sub-fertility. In Gordts, S. (ed.) *Current Status of Micromanipulation*, pp. 39–56. (Leuven: Drukkerij Nauwelaerts)

24. Gordts, S., Bassil, S., Pensis, M., Swinnen, K., Vercruyssen, M., Roziers, P., Thuyen, T., Campo, R. and Donnez, J. (1993). Subzonal insemination: treatment in cases of male subfertility? In Gordts, S. (ed.) *Current Status of Micromanipulation*, pp. 71–83. (Leuven: Drukkerij Nauwelaerts)

25. Fishel, S., Timson, J., Lisi, F. and Rinaldi, L. (1992). The evaluation of 225 patients undergoing subzonal insemination for the procurement of fertilisation in-vitro. *Fertil. Steril.*, **57**, 840–9

26. Wolf, J.P.H., Ducot, B., Kunstmann, J.M., Frydman, R. and Jouannet, P. (1992). Influence of sperm parameters on outcome of subzonal insemination in the case of previous IVF failure. *Hum. Reprod.*, **7**, 1407–13

27. Fishel, S., Timson, J., Antinori, S., Lisi, F. and Rinaldi, L. (1993). Subzonal insemination and zona breaching techniques for assisted fertilisation. Fishel, S. and Symonds, E.M. (eds.) *Gamete and Embryo Micromanipulation in Human Reproduction*, pp. 79–97. (London: Edward Arnold)

28. Sathananthan, A.H. (1994). Functional competence of abnormal spermatozoa. Fishel, S. (ed.) *Baillière's Obstetrics & Gynaecology – Micromanipulation Techniques*, pp. 141–56. (London: Baillière Tindall)

29. Van Steirteghem, A.C., Liu, J. and Joris, H. (1993). Higher success rate by intracytoplasmic sperm injection than by subzonal insemination. A report of a second series of 300 consecutive treatment cycles. *Hum. Reprod.*, **8**, 1055–60

30. Van Steirteghem, A.C., Nagy, Z., Joris, H., Lui, J., Staessen, C., Smitz, J., Wisanto, A. and Devroey, P. (1993). High fertilisation and implantation rates after intracytoplasmic sperm injection. *Hum. Reprod.*, **8**, 1061–6

31. Fishel, S., Timson, J., Lisi, F., Jacobson, M., Rinaldi, L. and Gobertz, L.

(1994). Micro-assisted fertilisation in patients who have failed sub-zonal insemination. *Hum. Reprod.*, **9**, 501–5

32. Gianaroli, L., Magli, M.C., Ferraretti, A.P., Fiorentino, A., Fortini, D. and Felicini, E. (1993). Outcome of new strategies for moderate and extreme male factor infertility. In Gordts, S. (ed.) *Current Status of Micromanipulation*, pp. 59–68. (Leuven: Drukkerij Nauwelaerts)

33. Hamberger, L., Sjörgen, A., Lundin, K., Söderlund, B. and Nilsson, L. (1993). Microfertilisation techniques – Scandinavian experience. In Gordts, S. (ed.) *Current Status of Micromanipulation*, pp. 85–9 (Leuven: Drukkerij Nauwelaerts)

34. Sathananthan, A.H., Ng, S.-C., Bongso, A. and Ratnam, S.S. (1993). Sperm micro-injection and micro-fertilisation. In Fishel, S.B. and Symonds, E.M. (eds.) *Gamete and Embryo Micromanipulation in Human Reproduction*, pp. 61–78. (London: Edward Arnold)

35. Fishel, S.B., Green, S., Dowell, K., Thornton, S., McDermott, H., Lisi, F., Rinaldi, L., Jacobson, M. and Gobetz, L. (1994). Fifty-nine cases of extreme male factor infertility – immotile sperm, Kartagener syndrome, globozoospermia, spermatogenic arrest, testicular sperm – treated by SUZI / ICSI. *Scientia*, **3**, 2

36. Ng, S.-C., Bongso, T.A., Liow, S.L., Montag, M., Tok, V. and Ratnam, S.S. (1993). New advances in micromanipulation: applications for treatment of the severe male factor patient. In Fishel, S.B. and Symonds, E.M. (eds.) *Gamete and Embryo Micromanipulation in Human Reproduction*, pp. 130–2. (London: Edward Arnold)

37. Ogura, A., Junichiro, M. and Yanagimachi, R. (1994). Birth of normal young after electrofusion of mouse oocytes with round spermatids. *Dev. Biol.*, **91**, 7460–2

38. Tadir, Y., Wright, W.H., Vafa, O., Liaw, L.H., Asch, R.H. and Berns, M.W. (1989). Micromanipulation of sperm by a laser generated optical trap. *Fertil. Steril.*, **52**, 870–3

39. Tadir, Y., Neev, J. and Burns, M.W. (1994). Laser microbeams for gamete manipulation. In Fishel, S. (ed.) *Ballière's Obstetrics & Gynaecology – Micromanipulation Techniques*, pp. 117–25. (London: Ballière Tindall)

40. Tadir, Y. (1994). Microsurgical fertilization world survey 1993. In Fishel, S. (ed.) *Ballières Obstetrics and Gynaecology – Micromanipulation Techniques*, pp. 197–203. (London: Ballière Tindall)

10

Cryopreservation: sperm and embryos – results in question

P. L. Matson, G. Horne, F. Hamer, S.A.C. Hotchkies, E.H.E. Pease, S.A. Troup and B.A. Lieberman

CRYOPRESERVATION OF GAMETES AND EMBRYOS

The cryopreservation of gametes and embryos involves storage at low temperatures, and includes both freezing[1,2] (by changing the liquid to a solid) and vitrification[3,4] (by conversion of the liquid to a glass, i.e. non-crystalline solid). The use of cryopreservation in clinical practice has enabled pregnancies to be achieved following the thawing of sperm[5], oocytes[6] and embryos[7,8]. However, the cryopreservation of oocytes presents many difficulties[9] and little progress has been made until recently[10]. On the other hand, the cryopreservation of sperm and embryos for clinical use is becoming widespread, and efforts are now being made to further simplify the protocols for both sperm[11,12] and embryos[13].

CLINICAL NEED

Sperm

Cryopreservation of semen is the only means by which it may be stored for long periods of time. This is now utilized widely as a method of quarantining donated semen. Since the transmission of human immuno-deficiency virus (HIV) by donor insemination to a recipient[14], both the American Fertility Society[15] and the British Andrology Society[16] have introduced guidelines recommending a minimum period of 6 months' quarantine. After this time, the donor can then be re-assessed for the presence of HIV antibodies and, if sero-conversion has not taken place, the semen used.

The long-term storage of semen by cryopreservation is also of benefit for men about to undergo cancer therapy before the illness affects semen quality adversely[17]. Given that the cancer requires treatment to begin as soon as possible, semen may be collected after the commencement of chemotherapy and pregnancies achieved[18]. However, the risk of genetic damage to the sperm by either chemotherapy[19] or radiotherapy[20] would suggest that the semen collection should be restricted to the period prior to treatment.

The storage of semen prior to vasectomy has been indicated[21] and is feasible. Nevertheless, it is not available widely, as many surgeons prefer not to have this back-up facility in order that patients may commit themselves fully to the operation. Semen may also be stored for patients undergoing treatment by assisted conception techniques and who are unable to provide a sample on the day of insemination because of psychological difficulties or because of absence due to work commitments, and also for those men with spinal injuries who require vibratory stimulation or electro-ejaculation[22]. However, the stockpiling of poor-quality semen by cryopreservation from patients for use at a later date has not proven of value because of poor post-thaw survival and the persistent poor functional qualities of the individual sperm cells[21].

Embryos

The cryopreservation and storage of embryos remaining after transfer in an *in vitro* fertilization (IVF) programme has proved useful worldwide[23] by allowing patients the opportunity to become pregnant by the subsequent replacement of thawed embryos, without the need for repeat ovarian stimulation and oocyte recovery. A similar benefit is seen for patients undergoing gamete intrafallopian transfer (GIFT) whereby the supernumerary oocytes are fertilized and frozen in the same unit[24], or fertilized during intra-vaginal culture and transport to a regional freezing facility[25].

A significant risk to patients undergoing ovarian stimulation for IVF/GIFT is the possible development of ovarian hyperstimulation syndrome. The elective cryopreservation of all embryos in such patients can avoid the transfer of embryos and the need for luteal support, and results in the reduced severity of symptoms without reducing the cumulative chance of pregnancy[26].

A further application of embryo cryopreservation can be seen in the operation of an ovum donation programme. The fertilization and subsequent storage of these oocytes removes the need for synchronization of donor and recipient[27] so that embryos may be thawed at the convenience of the recipient. Moreover, this approach also allows the quarantine of fertilized donated oocytes[28] to minimize the risk of HIV transmission, in exactly the same way as with donated semen. This use may well grow in importance as confidence in the freezing methods increases and greater attention is given to this aspect of ovum donation.

LEGISLATION

Increasing concern over the ethical and moral aspects of work involving human gametes and embryos has resulted in some countries introducing legislation to regulate the application of reproductive technology[29]. The UK was the first to introduce wide-reaching regulation by the introduction of the Human Fertilisation and Embryology Act (1990)[30] to cover the storage of gametes and the creation, storage and clinical use of embryos. This forms the statutory framework within which centres must work, and the activities using gametes and embryos are governed by the Act and authorized by the means of a licensing system administered by the appointed Human Fertilisation and Embryology Authority. In essence, three kinds of licence exist, namely those for treatment, storage and research. The range of activities undertaken by licensed centres in the UK during 1993 is given in Table 1, showing the proportion that freeze embryos and use frozen sperm for donor insemination. Germany has since introduced legislation covering these aspects[31].

Sperm

The Human Fertilisation and Embryology Act has had a major impact on the cryopreservation of semen in the UK. Men donating semen for use in

Table 1   The number of activities authorized by the Human Fertilisation and Embryology Act (1990) and carried out by the 109 licensed units during 1993

Activity	*Number of centres*
In vitro fertilization	62 (57%)
Donor insemination	93 (85%)
Research	16 (15%)
Egg donation	45 (41%)
Embryo freezing	49 (45%)

a donor insemination programme are now screened according to the British Andrology Society guidelines[16] for infectious diseases and genetic disorders, and the semen has to be quarantined for a minimum of 6 months to allow repeat testing of the donor for HIV. This semen can be stored for a maximum of 10 years only, after which it should be destroyed, and semen from any one donor can only produce ten viable pregnancies. The legal status of children born as a consequence of donor insemination has now been clarified, and they are regarded as being legitimate providing that consent was obtained from the male partner for the insemination to take place. Details of all donors, recipients and children are kept at a central registry, and anonymity between donor and recipient/offspring has been assured[32].

The storage of patients' semen is also governed by the Act, and the major impact has been in the length of time that semen from men with impending reduced fertility (e.g. cancer therapy, vasectomy) can be stored. To allow reasonable time for the semen to be used to inseminate the man's partner, the Act permits storage until he reaches 55 years of age. Providing appropriate consent is given, the semen may be used after the death of the man.

Embryos

The creation and cryopreservation of embryos is also governed by the Act, with an 'embryo' defined as an egg in the process of fertilization.

For practical purposes, this is taken as being from the time of insemination, as the fertilization process is said to begin with the first possible binding of sperm to the oocyte, and so the cryopreservation of embryos at either the pronucleate or early cleavage stages is bound by the Act. This contrasts with the situation in Germany, where the freezing of embryos is not permitted, but an embryo is defined as any fertilized human oocyte after that time at which the pronuclei have fused (i.e. after cleavage, for practical purposes). This means that pronucleate embryos may be cryopreserved without legislative control.

Embryos are allowed to be stored for a maximum of 5 years in the UK from the time of the introduction of the Act on 1 August 1991 or the date of freezing, whichever is the later. However, thought must be given to the fate of those embryos in advance of the storage deadline, and it is likely that the obligatory disposal of such embryos after the deadline will be problematical[33].

SURVIVAL FOLLOWING CRYOPRESERVATION

Spermatozoa

The majority of protocols employed in the freezing of sperm use media containing glycerol as the cryoprotectant[34]. The choice of freezing protocol appears important for the optimization of survival rates, in terms of the cryoprotective medium used[34] and the method of addition to the semen[35]. The two most commonly used protocols use medium containing glycerol only[36] or supplemented with egg yolk and citrate[34], although the cryoprotectant may often prove toxic to the sperm[37]. Freezing is usually achieved by cooling the straws or ampoules of semen in nitrogen vapour, although this can lead to variable cooling rates and poorer survival of sperm, compared to controlled freezing using a machine[38].

Assessment of the post-thaw survival of sperm is usually fairly demanding, with progressive motility of the sperm needing to be maintained, rather than just viability. Nevertheless, the likelihood of achieving a pregnancy with a sample after thawing can be difficult to assess, as is shown by Figure 1, since there appeared to be no difference in the range of post-thaw survival rates for two semen donors, and yet one achieved no

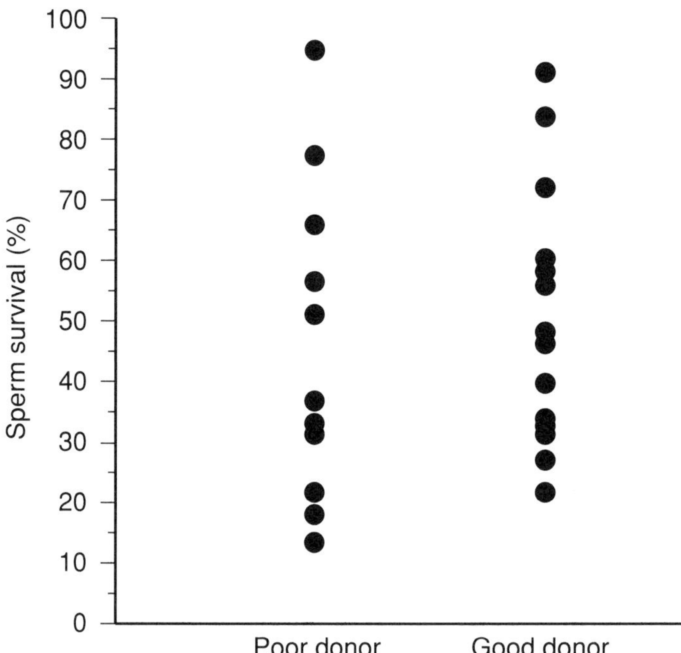

Figure 1 The post-thaw survival of sperm from two donors, one with a poor pregnancy rate and one achieving a good pregnancy rate

pregnancies and the other had a pregnancy rate > 20% per insemination. The post-thaw longevity of those sperm surviving the freeze–thaw procedure is often affected adversely[39,40], and this may be important in determining the effectiveness of samples used for insemination.

Embryos

The cryopreservation of human embryos can be undertaken at various stages of development using different cryoprotective agents, as reviewed by Ashwood-Smith[41]. In essence, embryos are usually frozen slowly and thawed rapidly, with the cryoprotectants for pronucleate, early cleavage embryos and blastocysts being propanediol[42], dimethylsulphoxide (DMSO)[43] or propanediol[44] and glycerol[45], respectively. The criteria for survival after thawing are very different for the three stages[46], and are summarized below.

Pronucleate embryos

Pronucleate embryos are cryopreserved as a single cell with pronuclei, the day after insemination. Upon thawing, they should have clear cytoplasm, an intact zona pellucida, and be shown to be capable of cleavage following overnight culture.

Early cleavage embryos

Early cleavage embryos are cryopreserved at any stage between 2–8 cells on either day 2 or 3 after insemination. After thawing, the embryo should have ≥50% of its blastomeres viable and the zona pellucida intact. However, embryos with just one or two viable blastomeres are capable of generating a pregnancy[47], albeit at a reduced rate, presumably because of the totipotency of the individual cells at this stage[48]. Early cleavage embryos are usually transferred on the same day as thawed, without further culture.

Blastocysts

Blastocysts are cryopreserved at the expanded stage. After thawing, the blastocoele should re-expand, usually after overnight culture, and there should be minimal areas of necrosis within the embryo, although this is often difficult to quantify.

Embryo survival

Survival rates of 60–70% per embryo after thawing are commonly reported. This is illustrated in Table 2 for the results obtained at St Mary's Hospital, Manchester, UK, and Manchester Fertility Services, UK, where the survival of pronucleate and early cleavage embryos was similar. Of those couples having embryos thawed, the majority were able to have at least one embryo transferred, although this high proportion is obviously related to the number of embryos cryopreserved initially for each couple. It appears that the successful survival of early cleavage embryos is inversely related to the number of cells present in the embryo at freezing, with the surface area of the blastomeres an important factor[49]. The initial quality of the embryo, though, is one of the major determinants of the suitability for transfer after thawing, such that the poor-quality embryos look even worse after the rigours of the freeze–thaw process[48,50]. The survival rate of

Table 2 The survival of human embryos following cryopreservation at St Mary's Hospital, Manchester and Manchester Fertility Services, UK and the proportion of couples having at least one embryo replaced

| | *Embryo stage at cryopreservation* | |
	pronucleate	*early cleavage*
Embryos thawed	2194	907
Embryos survived	1491 (67%)	592 (66%)
Couples	463	240
Thaws	788	301
Transfers	785 (99%)	270 (90%)

expanded blastocysts is said to compare favourably with that of early cleavage embryos[51], although blastocyst freezing is not offered widely because of the low rate of blastocyst formation in culture[52,53]. Whilst the use of co-culture systems may well improve the efficiency with which human blastocysts can be grown in the laboratory[54], the main impetus behind this approach would be to identify and discard those embryos which would be unlikely to grow in the body, and to increase the pregnancy rate per transfer by performing fewer fruitless transfers. However, it is doubtful whether any further pregnancies would be achieved by the extended culture and subsequent transfer of blastocysts, in women that otherwise would not have done so with cryopreservation at the pronucleate or early cleavage stage.

PREGNANCY RATES USING CRYOPRESERVED SPERMATOZOA AND EMBRYOS

The ultimate clinical reason for the cryopreservation of gametes and embryos must be to achieve a pregnancy as a result of their subsequent use. The pregnancy rates reported are often variable, and it is often difficult to assess whether the effects of poor technique or fundamental limitations of the methodology are contributing to lower success rates.

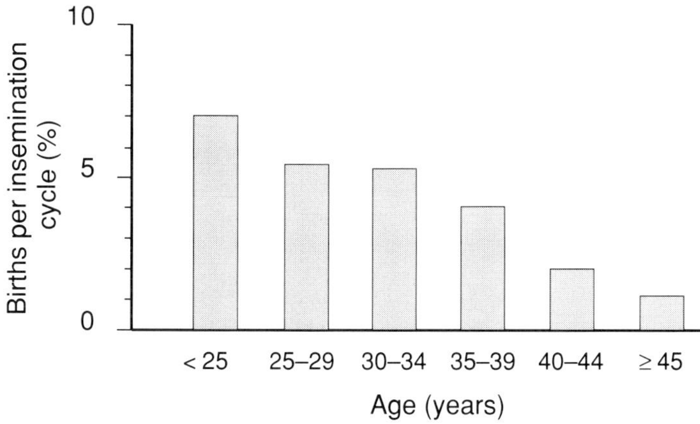

Figure 2 The birth rates per insemination cycle according to the woman's age at treatment by donor insemination. (Data from ref. 55)

Spermatazoa

The Human Fertilization and Embryology Act (1990) made obligatory the collection of pregnancy data in the UK following the use of donated semen. The data for donor insemination undertaken during 1992 in the UK[55] showed an overall live birth rate of 5.0% per insemination cycle, with the results showing a gradual decline with advancing age of the woman being treated (Figure 2). These results are particularly disappointing when one considers that the vast majority of cases would have had a severe male factor present, and that substitution of the male partner's semen with good-quality semen should have overcome the major contributory factor to the couple's infertility. A similar low pregnancy rate was observed in the Donor Insemination programme at St Mary's Hospital, Manchester, reaching a nadir in 1992 (Table 3). It is interesting to note that the introduction of monitoring in some patients with urinary luteinizing hormone (LH) kits during the beginning of 1993, compared with the timing of insemination based only on the length of the menstrual cycle, resulted in an increase in the number of pregnancies achieved. However, the largest increase was seen with the wholesale introduction of serum LH monitoring and intrauterine insemination. By performing a single intrauterine insemination of sperm prepared using Percoll® on the day after the onset of the LH surge, a pregnancy rate approaching

Table 3 The evolution of the donor insemination programme at St Mary's Hospital, Manchester. LH, luteinizing hormone

Period	Insemination method	Timing of insemination	Pregnancies per insemination	
Jan.–Dec. 1989	vaginal	menses	40 / 808	(5.0%)
Jan.–Dec. 1990	vaginal	menses	26 / 541	(4.8%)
Jan.–Dec. 1991	vaginal	menses	15 / 442	(3.4%)
Jan.–Dec. 1992	vaginal	menses	7 / 566	(1.2%)
Jan.–July 1993	vaginal	menses / LH	25 / 362	(6.9%)
Aug. 1993–April 1994	intrauterine	LH	101 / 508	(19.9%)

20% per insemination cycle was achieved and sustained. This compares favourably with the fecundity seen in the fertile population[56]. As this was a modification in the routine management of patients rather than a prospective study, it is impossible to know the relative contributions of either of these changes. However, the patients and bank of donors were as before, suggesting that the earlier low pregnancy rate was restricted by technical limitations connected with the nature and timing of the insemination procedure.

The value of intrauterine insemination in improving donor insemination pregnancy rates remains unclear, with increased success over and above intravaginal / intracervical insemination being seen by some workers[57,58] but not others[59]. One advantage that the intrauterine route may have is in the performance of the insemination close to ovulation by bypassing the cervical mucus which becomes increasingly impermeable to sperm after the LH surge[60], given the reduced life-span of frozen–thawed sperm[39,40]. The introduction of IVF[61] and GIFT[62] in the treatment of patients who have failed with a course of donor insemination may well give improved results, despite the increased invasive nature of the treatment.

Whatever the reasons behind the poor results obtained generally with donor insemination, methods to improve results should be considered by all concerned in the running of assisted conception programmes.

Table 4 Live birth rates following the transfer of frozen–thawed embryos at St Mary's Hospital, Manchester and Manchester Fertility Services

Replacement cycle	Pronucleate embryos		Early cleavage embryos	
Natural cycle	64 / 433	(14.8%)	23 / 165	(13.9%)
Hormone replacement therapy cycle	64 / 463	(13.8%)	13 / 140	(9.3%)
Total	128 / 896	(14.3%)	36 / 305	(11.8%)

Embryos

The value of an embryo cryopreservation programme in storing and subsequently using embryos from IVF treatment cycles, that would otherwise be unavailable for use by the patient, is constantly being demonstrated in the literature[63]. The results obtained at St Mary's Hospital, Manchester, and Manchester Fertility Services are given in Table 4 and illustrate the results commonly achieved. In our hands, there is little difference in pregnancy rates achieved, whether the embryos were cryopreserved at the pronucleate or early cleavage stages, or replaced into natural cycles or cycles in which the endometrium is stimulated with exogenous steroids[25]. In the UK overall, according to statistics gathered by the Human Fertilisation and Embryology Authority[55], 231 live births occurred following the transfer of frozen–thawed embryos in 2150 cycles during 1992, resulting in a live birth rate of 10.7% per embryo transfer.

The beneficial effect of the projected cumulative pregnancy rates of the subsequent transfer of frozen–thawed embryos from the original IVF cycle has been stated[64]. This mirrors what was actually seen in our Manchester units when the cumulative pregnancy rate of the frozen embryo transfers was added on to the original IVF cycle, as shown in Figure 3, where over 50% couples will achieve a pregnancy from a single oocyte recovery followed by transfer of fresh embryos in that cycle and by three transfers of frozen–thawed embryos. This cumulative pregnancy rate compares favourably with the results of the donor insemination programme using cryopreserved sperm shown in the same graph. Pregnancy rates of 10–20% per transfer of frozen-thawed embryos are

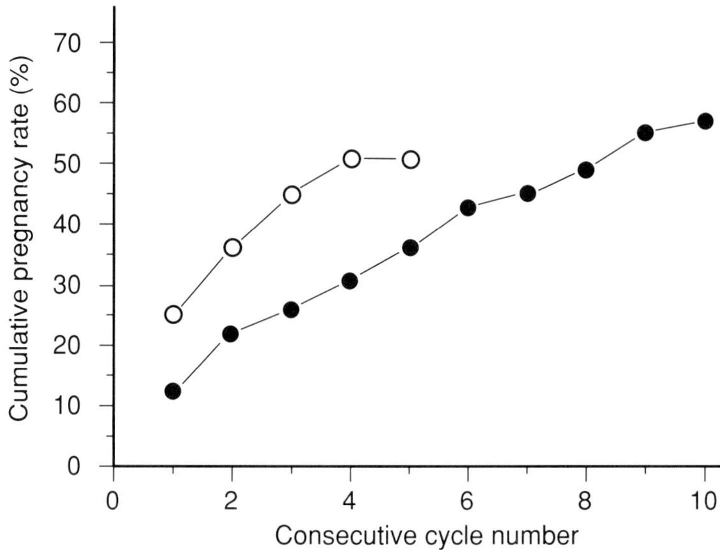

Figure 3 The cumulative pregnancy rate for vaginal insemination using donor sperm (●), and for *in vitro* fertilization (IVF) followed by the subsequent transfer of frozen–thawed embryos from that original IVF cycle (O)

often reported[2,23,64–66]. The effect of different factors upon the pregnancy rates has been examined, but the major determinant appears to be the quality of the embryos at the time of freezing[67].

The implantation rate of individual embryos is often measured by comparing the number of babies born with the number of embryos transferred, although assumptions are made about the lack of monozygotic multiple pregnancies and the endometrium having no limiting effect on the implantation. Nevertheless, the implantation rates obtained at the Manchester units are given in Table 5. There was a slightly lower implantation rate when compared to the fresh embryos from the original cycle, although it did not reach significance. Implantation rates of between 5–15% per embryo have been reported elsewhere[2,50,64].

Concern has been expressed regarding the safety of embryo cryoprotectants and their long-term genetic effects[68]. Whilst we should continue to monitor the progress of children born from the transfer of frozen–thawed embryos, there is no evidence for a 'lack of safety for patients or their potential children'[55], and the children appear similar at birth to IVF children in general[69].

Table 5 The implantation rate per egg or embryo after replacement at St Mary's Hospital, Manchester and Manchester Fertility Services (IVF, *in vitro* fertilization; GIFT, gamete intrafallopian transfer)

	Treatment cycle			
	IVF	*GIFT*	*Pronucleate embryos*	*Early cleavage embryos*
Cycles	683	215	785	270
Egg/embryos replaced	1761	774	1491	596
Babies	175	54	112	37
Implantation rate	9.9%	6.9%	7.5%	5.6%

CONCLUSIONS

The cryopreservation of sperm and embryos has tremendous clinical value, and reliable methods to cryopreserve oocytes would further help improve clinical services. Sperm from donors may be quarantined, whilst sperm from patients may be stored prior to cancer therapy or in cases where semen production is difficult. However, further work is clearly needed to improve the overall pregnancy rates following donor insemination. Embryo cryopreservation enables supernumerary embryos from GIFT and IVF cycles to be stored and used subsequently, thereby maximizing the chance of pregnancy per oocyte recovery. The provision of embryo cryopreservation facilities at all IVF units should be encouraged.

ACKNOWLEDGEMENTS

The help given by all the staff in the Department of Reproductive Medicine, St Mary's Hospital, Manchester and at Manchester Fertility Services is greatly appreciated.

REFERENCES

1. Watson, P.F., Critser, J.K. and Mazur, P. (1992). Sperm preservation: fundamental cryobiology and practical implications. In Templeton, A.A. and Drife, J.O. (eds.) *Infertility*, pp.101–14. (London: Springer-Verlag)

2. Friedler, S., Giudice, L.C. and Lamb, E.J. (1988). Cryopreservation of embryos and ova. *Fertil Steril.*, **49**, 743–64

3. Polge, C., Smith, A.W. and Parkes, A.S. (1949). Revival of spermatozoa after vitrification and dehydration at low temperatures. *Nature (London)*, **164**, 666

4. Rall, W.F. and Fahy, G.M. (1984). Ice-free cryopreservation of mouse embryos at −196°C by vitrification. *Nature (London)*, **313**, 573–5

5. Bunge, R.G. and Sherman, J. (1953). Fertilizing capacity of frozen human spermatozoa. *Nature (London)*, **172**, 767–8

6. Chen, C. (1986). Pregnancy after human oocyte cryopreservation. *Lancet*, **1**, 884–6

7. Trounson, A. and Mohr, L.R. (1983). Human pregnancy following cryopreservation, thawing and transfer of an eight-cell embryo. *Nature (London)*, **305**, 707–9

8. Zeilmaker, G.H., Alberda, A.Th., Van Gent, I., Rifkmans, C.M.P.M. and Drogendijk, A.C. (1984). Two pregnancies following transfer of intact frozen–thawed embryos. *Fertil. Steril.*, **2**, 293–6

9. Whittingham, D.G. and Carroll, J.G. (1992). Cryopreservation of mammalian oocytes. In Templeton, A.A. and Drife, J.O. (eds.) *Infertility*, pp.253–61. (London: Springer-Verlag)

10. Gook, D.A., Osborn, S.M., Bourne, H. and Johnston, W.I.H. (1994). Fertilization of human oocytes following cryopreservation: normal karyotypes and absence of stray chromosomes. *Hum. Reprod.*, **9**, 684–91

11. Kremer, J., Dijkhuis, J.R.H. and Jager, S. (1987). A simplified method for freezing and storage of human semen. *Fertil. Steril.*, **47**, 838–42

12. Morroll, D.R., Matson, P.L., Troup, S.A., Izzard, H., Prior, J.R., Burslem, R.W. and Lieberman, B.A. (1990). The cryopreservation of donor semen by a simplified method: use in an IVF and GIFT programme. *Int. J. Androl.*, **13**, 352–60

13. Trounson, A., Peura, A. and Kirby, C. (1987). Ultrarapid freezing: a new low-cost and effective method of embryo cryopreservation. *Fertil. Steril.*, **48**, 843–50

14. Stewart, G., Tyler, J.P.P., Cunningham, A.L., Barr, J.A., Driscoll, G.L., Gold, J. and Lamont, B.J. (1985). Transmission of human T-cell lymphotropic virus type III (HTLV-III) by artificial insemination by donor. *Lancet*, **2**, 581–4

15. American Fertility Society (1993). Guidelines for gamete donation: 1993. *Fertil. Steril.*, **59** (Suppl. 1)

16. Barratt, C.L.R., Matson, P.L. and Holt, W. (1993). British Andrology Society guidelines for the screening of semen donors for donor insemination. *Hum Reprod.*, **8**, 1521–3

17. Hendry, W.F.F., Stedronska, J., Jones, C.R., Blackmore, C.A., Barrett, A. and Peckham, M.J. (1983). Semen analysis in testicular cancer and Hodgkin's disease: pre- and post-treatment findings and implications for cryopreservation. *Br. J. Urol.*, **55**, 769–73

18. Carson, S.A., Gentry, W.L., Smith, A.L. and Buster, J.E. (1991). Feasibility of semen collection and cryopreservation during chemotherapy. *Hum. Reprod.*, **6**, 992–4

19. Meistrich, M.L. (1993). Potential genetic risks using semen collected during chemotherapy. *Hum. Reprod.*, **8**, 8–10

20. Rousseaux, S., Sele, B., Cozzi, J. and Chevret, E. (1993). Immediate rearrangements of human sperm chromosomes following *in-vivo* irradiation. *Hum. Reprod.*, **8**, 903–7

21. Schoysman, R., Schoysman-Deboeck, A., van Roosendaal, E., Grijp, L., Segal-Bertin, G. and Van Der Zwalman, P. (1990). Cryopreservation of sperm and its clinical applications. In Asch, R.H., Balmaceda, J.P. and Johnston, I. (eds.) *Gamete Physiology*, pp.199–208. (Norwell: Serono Symposia)

22. Padron, O.F., Brackett, N.L., Weizman, M.S. and Lynne, C.M. (1994). Semen of spinal cord injured men freezes reliably. *J. Androl.*, **15**, 266–9

23. Van Steirteghem, A.C. and van den Abbeel, E. (1988). Survey on cryopreservation. *Ann. N. Y. Acad. Sci.*, **541**, 571–4

24. Van Steirteghem, A.C., van den Abbeel, E., Camus, M., Van Waesberghe, L., Braeckmans, P., Khan, I., Nijs, M., Smitz, J., Staessen, C., Wisanto, A. and Devroey, P. (1987). Cryopreservation of human embryos obtained after gamete intra-Fallopian transfer and / or *in-vitro* fertilization. *Hum. Reprod.*, **2**. 593–8

25. Critchlow, J.D., Matson, P.L., Killick, S. and Lieberman, B.A. (1992). Pregnancy following intra-vaginal embryo transportation. *Br. J. Obstet. Gynaecol.*, **99**, 259–60

26. Wada, I., Matson, P.L., Troup, S.A., Hughes, S., Buck, P. and Lieberman, B.A. (1992). Outcome of treatment subsequent to the elective cryopreservation of all embryos from women at risk of the ovarian hyperstimulation syndrome. *Hum. Reprod.*, **7**, 962–6

27. Salat-Baroux, J., Cornet, D., Alvarez, S., Antoine, J.M., Tibi, C., Mandelbaum, J. and Plachot, M. (1988). Pregnancies after replacement of frozen–thawed embryos in a donation programme. *Fertil. Steril.*, **49**, 817–21

28. Hamer, F., Matson, P.L., Horne, G., Troup, S.A., Buck, P., Hotchkies, S. and Lieberman, B.A. (1992). The quarantine of fertilised donated oocytes. *J. Reprod. Fertil. Abstr. Series*, **10**, 52

29. Gunning, J. and English, V. (1993). *Human In Vitro fertilization*, (Aldershot: Dartmouth Publishing)

30. British Acts of Parliament (1990). Human Fertilisation and Embryology Act, 1990. Chapter 37, pp.1–39. (London: Her Majesty's Stationery Office)

31. Beier, H.M. and Beckman, J.O. (1991). German Embryo Protection Act (October 24th, 1990): Gesetz zum Schutz von Embryonen (Embryonen-shutzgesetz-ESchG). *Hum. Reprod.*, **6**, 605–6

32. Bottomley, V. (1991). Hansard, 3rd May

33. Shenfield, F., Matson, P.L., Horne, G., Hamer, F., Lieberman, B.A. and Steele, S.J.S. (1993). The statutory limit for embryo storage in the UK: a potential problem for 1996. *Dispatches*, **4**, 8–9

34. Weidel, L. and Prins, G.S. (1987). Cryosurvival of human spermatozoa frozen in eight different buffer systems. *J. Androl.*, **8**, 41–7

35. Mahadevan, M. and Trounson, A.O. (1993). Effects of cryoprotective media and dilution methods on the preservation of human spermatozoa. *Andrologia*, **15**, 355–66

36. Mahadevan, M., Trounson, A.O. and Leeton, J. (1983). Successful use of human semen cryobanking for *in vitro* fertilisation. *Fertil. Steril.*, **40**, 340–3

37. McLaughlin, E.A., Ford, W.C.L. and Hull, M.G.R. (1992). The contribution of the toxicity of a glycerol-egg yolk-citrate cryopreservative to the decline in human sperm motility during cryopreservation. *J. Reprod. Fertil.*, **95**, 749–54

38. McLaughlin, E.A., Ford, W.C.L. and Hull, M.G.R. (1990). A comparison of the freezing of human semen in the uncirculated vapour above liquid nitrogen and in a commercial semi-programmable freezer. *Hum. Reprod.*, **5**, 724–8

39. Keel, B.A. and Black, J.B. (1980). Reduced motility longevity in thawed human spermatozoa. *Arch. Androl.*, **4**, 213–5

40. Critser, J.K., Arneson, B.W., Aaker, D.V., Huse-Benda, A.R. and Ball, G.D. (1987). Cryopreservation of human spermatozoa. II. Post-thaw chronology of motility and of zona-free hamster ova penetration. *Fertil. Steril.*, **47**, 980–4

41. Ashwood-Smith, M.J. (1986). The cryopreservation of human embryos. *Hum. Reprod.*, **1**, 319–32

42. Lassalle, B., Testart, J. and Renard, J-P. (1985). Human embryo features that influence the success of cryopreservation with the use of 1,2 propanediol. *Fertil. Steril.*, **44**, 645–51

43. Cohen, J., Simons, R.F., Edwards, R.G., Fehilly, C.B. and Fishel, S.B.

(1985). Pregnancies following storage of expanding human blastocysts. *J. In Vitro Fertil. Embryo Transfer*, **2**, 59–64

44. Mohr, L. and Trounson, A.O. (1985). Cryopreservation of human embryos. *Ann. N. Y. Acad. Sci.*, **442**, 536–43

45. Troup, S.A., Matson, P.L., Critchlow, J.D., Morroll, D.R., Lieberman, B.A. and Burslem, R.W. (1990). Cryopreservation of human embryos at the pronucleate, early cleavage or expanded blastocyst stages. *Eur. J. Obstet. Gynaecol. Reprod. Biol.*, **38**, 133–9

46. Veiga, A., Calderon, G., Barri, P.N. and Coroleu, B. (1987). Pregnancy after the replacement of a frozen–thawed embryo with < 50% intact blastomeres. *Hum. Reprod.*, **2**, 321–3

47. Braude, P.R., Bolton, V. and Moore, S. (1988). Human gene expression first occurs between the four and eight cell stages of pre-implantation development. *Nature (London)*, **332**, 459–61

48. Mandelbaum, J., Junca, A.M., Plachot, M., Alnot, M.O., Alvarez, S., Debache, C., Salat-Baroux, J. and Cohen, J. (1987). Human embryo cryopreservation, extrinsic and intrinsic parameters of success. *Hum. Reprod.*, **2**, 709–15

49. Hartshorne, G.M., Wick, K., Elder, K. and Dyson, H. (1990). Effect of cell number at freezing upon survival and viability of cleaving embryos generated from stimulated IVF cycles. *Hum. Reprod.*, **5**, 857–61

50. Cohen, J., Simons, R.S., Fehilly, C.B. and Edwards, R.G. (1986). Factors affecting survival and implantation of cryopreserved human embryos. *J. In Vitro Fertil. Embryo Transfer*, **3**, 46–52

51. Fehilly, C.B., Cohen, J., Simons, R.F., Fishel, S.B. and Edwards, R.G. (1985). Cryopreservation of cleaving embryos and expanded blastocysts in the human: a comparative study. *Fertil. Steril.*, **44**, 638–44

52. Bolton, V.N., Hawes, S.M., Taylor, C.T. and Parsons, J.H. (1989). Development of spare human pre-implantation embryos *in-vitro*: an analysis of the correlates among gross morphology, cleavage rates, and development to blastocysts. *J. In Vitro Fertil. Embryo Transfer*, **6**, 30–5

53. Dokras, A., Sargent, I.L. and Barlow, D.H. (1994). Human blastocyst grading and chorionic gonadotropin secretion. In Mastroianni, L. Jr, Coelingh Bennink, H.J.T., Suzuki, S. and Vemer, H.M. (eds.) *Gamete and Embryo Quality*, pp.157–70. (Carnforth, UK: Parthenon Publishing)

54. Menezo, Y., Nicollet, B., Herbaut, N. and Andre, D. (1992). Freezing co-cultured human blastocysts. *Fertil. Steril.*, **58**, 977–80

55. Human Fertilisation and Embryology Authority (1994). Third Annual Report. (London: HFEA)

56. Clark, C. (1967) *Population Growth and Land Use*, (London: Macmillan)

57. Patton, P.E., Burry, K.A., Thurmond, A., Novy, M.J. and Wolf, D.P

(1992). Intra-uterine insemination outperforms intra-cervical insemination in a randomized controlled study with frozen donor semen. *Fertil. Steril.*, **57**, 559–64

58. Byrd, W., Bradshaw, K., Carr, B., Edman, C., Odam, J. and Ackerman, G. (1990). A prospective randomized study of pregnancy rates following intra-uterine and intra-cervical insemination using frozen donor semen. *Fertil.Steril.*, **53**, 521–7

59. Depypere, H.T., Gordts, S., Campo, R. and Comhaire, F. (1994). Methods to increase the success rate of artificial insemination with donor semen. *Hum. Reprod.*, **9**, 661–3

60. Moghissi, K.S., Syner, F.N. and Evans, T.N. (1972). A composite picture of the menstrual cycle. *Am. J. Obstet. Gynecol.*, **114**, 405–18

61. Kovacs, G.T., King, C., Rogers, P., Wood, C., Baker, H.W.G. and Yates, C. (1989). *In vitro* fertilization, a practical option after failed artificial insemination with donor sperm. *Reprod. Fertil. Dev.*, **1**, 383–6

62. Kovacs, G.T. and King, C. (1994). The use of gamete intra-Fallopian transfer with donor spermatozoa after failed donor insemination. *Hum. Reprod.*, **9**, 859–60

63. Wang, X.J., Ledger, W., Payne, D., Jeffrey, R. and Matthews C.D. (1994). The contribution of embryo cryopreservation to *in-vitro* fertilization/gamete intra-Fallopian transfer: 8 years experience. *Hum. Reprod.*, **9**, 103–9

64. Veeck, L.L., Amundson, C.H., Brothman, L.J., De Scisciolo, C., Maloney, M.K., Muasher, S.J. and Jones, H.W. Jr (1993). Significantly enhanced pregnancy rates per cycle through cryopreservation and thaw of pronuclear stage oocytes. *Fertil. Steril.*, **59**, 1202–7

65. Cohen, J., Kort, H.I., De Vane, G.W., Massey, J.B., Elsner, C.W., Turner, T.G. and Fehilly, C.B. (1988). Cryopreservation of zygotes and early cleaved human embryos. *Fertil. Steril.*, **49**, 283–9

66. Junca, A.M., Mandelbaum, J., Alnot, M.O., Plachot, M., Cohen, J. and Salat-Baroux, J. (1988). Factors involved in the success of human embryo freezing: does cryopreservation really improve the IVF results? *Ann. N. Y. Acad. Sci.*, **541**, 575–82

67. Schalkoff, M.E., Oskowitz, S.P. and Powers, R.D. (1993). A multi-factorial analysis of the pregnancy outcome in a successful embryo cryopreservation program. *Fertil. Steril.*, **59**, 1070–4

68. Winston, R.M.L. and Handyside, A.H. (1993). New challenges in human *in vitro* fertilization. *Science*, **260**, 932–6

69. Wada, I., Macnamee, M.C., Wick, K., Bradfield, J.M. and Brinsden, P.R. (1994). Birth characteristics and perinatal outcome of babies conceived from cryopreserved embryos. *Hum. Reprod.*, **9**, 543–6

Index